NATURAL WOMAN, NATURAL MENOPAUSE

MARCUS LAUX, N.D.,
AND CHRISTINE CONRAD

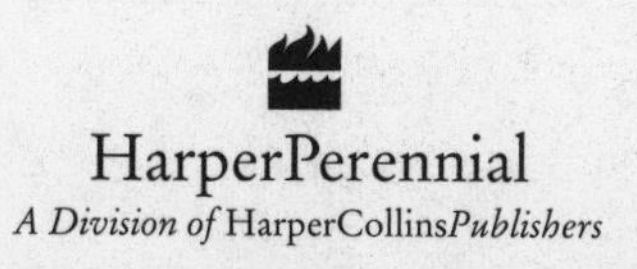

HarperPerennial
A Division of HarperCollins*Publishers*

This book should not be substituted for the personal care and attention of a qualified physician but rather should be used in conjunction with your physician's care and advice. Before beginning any new health, diet, or exercise program, you should always consult with a physician to be sure the new regimens are appropriate for your individual circumstances. The author and the publisher will not be responsible for any adverse effects resulting from the use or application of the information contained in this book.

A hardcover edition of this book was published in 1997 by HarperCollins Publishers.

HarperCollins books may be purchased for educational, business, or sales promotional use. For information please write: Special Markets Department, HarperCollins Publishers, Inc., 10 East 53rd Street, New York, NY 10022.

First HarperPerennial edition published 1998.

Designed by Alma Hochhauser Orenstein
Illustrations by Barbara Mindell

The Library of Congress has catalogued the hardcover edition as follows:

Laux, Marcus, 1952–
Natural woman, natural menopause / Marcus Laux and Christine Conrad. — 1st ed.
p. cm.
Includes bibliographical references and index.
ISBN 0-06-017341-6
1. Menopause—Complications—Alternative treatment.
2. Menopause—Hormone therapy. 3. Menopause—Popular works.
4. Naturopathy. I. Conrad, Christine, 1946– . II. Title.
RG186.L384 1997
618.1'75—dc21 96-30096

ISBN 0-06-092894-8 (pbk.)

03 04 05 06 ❖/RRD 20 19 18 17 16 15 14 13

CONTENTS

Appendixes

ACKNOWLEDGMENTS

We would like to thank Dr. Jesse Hanley, Dr. John Lee, Bruce MacFarland, Ph.D., Dr. Uzzi Reiss, Dr. Tori Hudson, Dr. Michael Murray, Dr. Zoe Wells, Dr. Barbara Beale, Dr. Carolyn DeMarco, Dr. Jamie Grifo, Dr. Alan Altman, Dr. T. Colin Campbell, Dr. Timothy Birdsall, Dr. James Jamison, Virginia Hopkins, Tim Sara, Mary Lloyd, Dr. Ray Peat, Dr. Donal Carter, Anne Ross, Dr. Corey Resnick, Dr. Jonathan Wright, Dr. Amber Ackerson, Dr. Peter Ellison, Sharon MacFarland, Gillian Ford, Gladys Warr, Dr. David Zava, John Kells, Dr. David Scheffrin, Shelly Schluter, Bill Conway, Dr. Guy Abraham, Kelley Sego, Elizabeth Retz, Scott Martin, Dr. Christiane Northrup, Dr. Mary James, Dr. Peter Wilhemmson, Bradley Norris and Catie Norris, Malibu Health & Rehabilitation, Barbara Mindell, Ann Gentry, Terry Lemerond, Phil Davis, J.D., Lynette Padwa.

Marla Ahlgrimm, R.Ph., Robert Harshbarger, R.Ph., George Roentsch, R.Ph., Gary Osborn, R.Ph., Tom Giacalone, R.Ph., Russell Gellis, R.Ph., Ron Miller, R.Ph., Mark Holzener, R.Ph., Joe Delk, R.Ph., Phil Hagerman, R.Ph., Robert Horwitz, R.Ph., Ken Hughes, R.Ph., Dave Mason, R.Ph., Evelyn Timmons, R.Ph., Tom Bader, R.Ph., Sam Georgio, R.Ph., Marx Gaines, R.Ph., George Malmer, R.Ph., Barry Mizer, R.Ph., Carol Peterson, R.Ph., Wally Simons, R.Ph., Peter Hueseman, R.Ph.

Also, our deepest thanks for the invaluable support of our agent, Jane Dystel. At HarperCollins, Janet Goldstein and Diane Reverand, who bought the book; our indispensable editor, Peternelle Van Arsdale; assistant editor Kristen Auclair; and our publicist Fran Rosencrantz.

I would especially like to thank all the women who shared personal stories with me and all the women who said, *You must write this book!* Lynette Padwa for her expert advice on the manuscript, Esther Margolis, Sherry Lansing, Kathy Eldon, Dawn Steel, Renee Schwartz, Davina Belling, Marsha Nasatir, Ellen Krass, Dr. Jesse Hanley, Dr. Uzzi Reiss, Tamara Berkovich, Lisa Inouye, Rebecca Floeter, Alison Cross, Barbara Corday, Jane Deknatel, Nancy Eddo, Jocelyne Eberstein, Fay Koliai, Patti Felker, Rosalind Ayres and Martin Jarvis, Shirley and George Perle, Dr. Daniel Stern and Nadia Stern, Clarice Rivers, Christina Wijaya, Rena Wolner, Mark Mawrence, Christine Macgenn, Jim Strohecker.

And for their great support during my illnesses: my sister, Diane Conrad, mother, Lucille Conrad, and nephews, Mark and Mathew Grein and Jerome Robbins.

Christine Conrad

I'm especially grateful for the support of Dr. Tori Hudson, Marla Ahlgrimm, Carol Peterson, Dr. Jesse Hanley, Emily Conrad Da'ouad, Helen Faraday, Joachim Lehmann, Mary Ann Liebert, Dr. David Field, Dr. Robert Schwartz, Donna Goldstein, J.D., Dr. Maureen Becker, Mary Reichwald, Jack Challem, Loren Israelsen, and Barbara Bassett.

The National College of Naturopathic Medicine, for the faith, the tools, and the degree that allows me to practice the medicine we all need for the twenty-first century.

Christine Macgenn, my enthusiastic and tireless research and editorial associate who kept the ball moving.

The deepest love and thanks that only a son can feel goes to my mom and dad.

And to my wife, Anita, for the love, joy, and commitment she brings me.

Marcus Laux

WHO IS THIS BOOK FOR?

The *two million* women coming into menopause each year.

The *forty million* presently in menopause and post-menopause.

The woman on HRT experiencing serious side effects.

The woman on HRT for more than five years, who is concerned about cancer risk.

The *one third of American women* who have been hysterectomized and are dependent on hormone replenishment.

Women who have refused help for their symptoms until now.

Women survivors of breast cancer, for whom HRT is very high-risk.

Women at high risk for heart disease and osteoporosis.

Women disillusioned by the treatment of women by the medical establishment.

Women confused by the conflicting information about the risks of HRT.

Young women with PMS, interested in how hormones work in their bodies.

Young women looking ahead.

Those who want to *remain* sexually vital, and those who want to be even *more* sexually vital.

Those who already know the power of natural medicine.

Those who want the gentler, safer, nontoxic effects of natural medicine.

Those who want to know about natural medicine, but don't know how to gain access to it.

Those who don't have time for endless experimentation.

Medical professionals who want a better way to treat their patients.

Patients who want to teach their doctors how to treat them better.

Those who want a *complete plan* that they can follow like a recipe.

Those who want to join the women who make the second part of life the best part of life.

A PERSONAL NOTE FROM CHRISTINE CONRAD

This is the book I couldn't find when, four years ago, I found myself on a search for an "alternative" source of estrogen. I was, at that time, in miserable physical condition. After a bout with peritonitis, followed by surgery for a bowel obstruction combined with a complete hysterectomy, I was beset by a period of illness brought on by complications of the operation. Adding to my difficulties, at a certain point gastrointestinal problems prevented me from continuing to ingest the Premarin I was automatically given after the operation. (A later test of my estrogen levels showed that I wasn't absorbing it very well anyway.) Stopping the Premarin brought on the symptoms of surgical menopause, which for me included hot flashes and joint pain. And not only were my estrogen levels very low, but a test showed that I was in an advanced stage of osteoporosis.

I was very scared, as I foresaw complications from the osteoporosis, and premature aging. I was desperate to find another way to get estrogen. My internist had no suggestions. Gynecologists I consulted told me that apart from Premarin and other synthetic estrogenic drugs produced by the major drug companies, there was no way to get the supplemental estrogen I needed. I was also led to believe that bone already lost to osteoporosis was lost forever. Though essentially abandoned to my fate by these practitioners, I persisted, because for one, I really didn't have a choice, and two, I just couldn't accept the finality of what they were telling me.

Almost all the published books on menopause at the time concentrated on the pros and cons of estrogen replacement, and those books advocating a "natural" menopause or dietary approach weren't clear or very trustworthy, presenting only a grabbag of natural remedies with trial and error possibilities that might take a lifetime.

Then, one day, a friend mentioned Dr. Marcus Laux, who was successfully treating women with plant-derived hormone preparations. Under his care, I began using a natural plant-derived estrogen/progesterone cream absorbed through the skin. I was initially skeptical that such a method would work, as back then I thought that somehow "medicine" only worked in "pill" form. In my case, taking estrogen/progesterone through the skin had the special virtue of bypassing my stomach and intestines—but I later came to understand that this method of absorption had the additional benefit of bypassing the liver, thereby eliminating the potential of liver disease, a known long-term side effect of the orally administered Premarin.

My improvement using this treatment was swift and complete. In less than three months, I no longer had joint pain, hot flashes, or any other menopausal symptoms, and there were no side effects. I also didn't experience the bloating and water retention that had accompanied my use of Premarin. After following the treatment plan for six months—which included the estrogen/progesterone cream absorbed through the skin; weight-resistance training; supplemental vitamins, minerals, and nutrients; and dietary changes—my estrogen levels were retested by my original internist. Not only had they improved, I now had the estrogen levels of a young menstruating female! And with no period! In addition, a further osteoporosis test showed that I had no evidence of the disease. The osteoporosis process had been completely reversed. As a further blessing, with Dr. Laux's help I was able to finally get a diagnosis and clear up the gastrointestinal problems—problems that, ironically, had prevented me from ingesting the Premarin in the first place.

I now feel great, look great, and appear years younger than my age.

When I think back over my years of illness, what do I remember as one of the worst symptoms? Confusion. *What do I do now? Should I take this drug? Am I being told the right thing? Does this doctor know what he is talking about? Should I talk to another doctor? What should I do next?* Your friends give you anecdoctal remedies. Try this, try that. Every day, you wake up in this confused state. When, after a seemingly well period, I got sick a second time with renewed malabsorption and other gastrointestinal problems, I was most upset about being back in this state of daily confusion.

With the success of my treatment, I began to wonder why it had been so difficult to find my way to it. I knew that there were legions of women out there without the option given to me. Not only had I found a safe, gentle, and effective way to replace estrogen, but it also appeared to be a *better* way, without the risk of cancer that came with the standard HRT treatment. I began to see the great blessing in my illness: Only through its crucible could I have been forced to look beyond the confusing standard prescriptions and dig deeply enough for a solution to my own hormone-related problems. Otherwise, I would have been one of the millions of women who upon reaching menopause would have to sift through the confusing information and perhaps never find the right solutions, or worse still, end up with the wrong solutions, which could jeopardize their long-term health.

My growing interest and curiosity in the subject led to talks with Dr. Laux during which I discovered that he had developed, exclusively through word of mouth, a large practice of women who were successfully following his treatment plan of using bio-identical plant hormone products. He is a member of a network of doctors who are pioneering this treatment for women—a group that includes a growing number of M.D.'s. I also found that in addition to the preformulated hormone creams I first used, I was astonished to learn that plant-derived estrogen and progesterone in a variety of standardized forms were available by prescription at compounding pharmacies across the country, and have been for well over a decade.

Until the onset of the peritonitis, I had been lucky in my health. My sudden plunge into illness had left me quite dismayed, to say the least, by my treatment by conventional medical practitioners. My experience was that if you didn't fit into standard disease protocols, if they couldn't treat you with their specified lists of drugs, you were simply abandoned. Worse still, these practitioners were all too quick to employ the "it's all in your head" charge. And no attention was paid to the overall *well-being* of the patient. Everything I had heard from other women about how badly they had been treated by their doctors was confirmed by my own experiences. Also, I discovered firsthand how little was really known about the effect of hormone fluctuations on a woman's health throughout her life.

We are children of Western medicine. Certainly, I was. I was conditioned to the idea that the way medicine is practiced in this country is the *only* way medicine can be practiced. When I was dabbling around with so-called "alternative" therapists in my desperate search for help, many of them struck me as undisciplined and untrustworthy. So when I first met Dr. Laux, I was stunned to discover that a medical discipline existed that combined the scientific training and professionalism of an M.D. with a concern for the patient's overall well-being and the use of healing substances that work with the body. I now know that naturopathic physicians are the only primary-care doctors in the United States who are fully trained in the use of effective medicinal plant remedies.

Further investigation into the "politics" of medicine began to shed light on how medical and pharmaceutical forces put their own interests ahead of the good health of women, and why they have not searched for safer alternatives to the HRT drugs, with their known side effects and long-term cancer potential.

And then I got angry.

At this time of my life, writing a book about menopause is probably not a great career move; my work as a screenwriter is thriving and I have many projects I'm excited about, but for me, none of these is as compelling or as vital as this book. One of the most important things I have learned is that a woman cannot afford to be passive when it comes to issues vital to her health and quality of life. She can't risk simply putting herself in the hands of others or accepting what is standard practice. In order to share my hard-won knowledge on hormones and how to stay youthful and full of vitality at midlife, I felt that Dr. Marcus Laux and I had to write *Natural Woman.*

We owed it to women everywhere.

A PERSONAL NOTE FROM DR. LAUX

I never anticipated writing a book about menopause. It was the women who came to my practice looking for help and seeking relief that focused me on the treatment of menopausal symptoms. Women today are led to believe that they have only one choice: "Do I take conventional hormone replacement therapy (HRT) and risk getting cancer, or do I avoid it and risk getting osteoporosis and heart disease?" If a woman follows today's conventional thinking, she is often asked to believe that all she needs is estrogen derived from horse urine and a couple of antacids with oyster shell calcium and she will be spared the problems of menopause. When she is not spared those problems, she wonders why. No one seems to be able to tell her.

This dilemma is occurring at a time when more and more women want a physician who understands and is trained in a more natural approach to their health care. A naturopathic physician is just this kind of doctor. Educated in the conventional medical sciences and technologies, naturopathic physicians are not orthodox medical doctors. We are specialists in natural medicine, uniquely schooled to treat disease and restore health by using natural therapies that include clinical nutrition; herbal, Asian, and Ayurvedic medicine; psychological counseling; exercise therapy; natural childbirth; physical medicine; homeopathy; and hydrotherapy. As a distinct health care profession, naturopathic medicine originated in Germany over 100 years ago, but its roots date back into medical antiquity.

I am a licensed naturopathic physician and I believe in the healing power of nature. I believe my job is to help nature do her job by removing the obstacles to healing, and by nourishing, stimulating, and strengthening the body's immune and repair systems. I believe you are more than your body—that your mind, body, and spirit are inextricably one, inseparable. If you are to achieve lasting, vital health, all aspects of your being need to be cared for and loved. While even those patients who use only conventional doctors are coming to realize this link between mind, body, and spirit, there is still a bias among many in the medical community against any medical discipline or practitioner they would term "alternative" even if they are M.D.'s. This bias is changing as the alternative becomes more and more accepted as part of the "mainstream."

As with all modern primary care doctors, naturopathic physicians are trained in medical schools accredited by a council recognized by the United States Department of Education. In North America there are four recognized naturopathic medical schools: National College in Portland, Oregon; Bastyr University in Seattle, Washington; Southwest College in Scottsdale, Arizona; and Ontario College in Ontario, Canada. The naturopathic physician earns the degree of Doctor of Naturopathic Medicine (N.D.) upon graduating from four years of residential, graduate-level, naturopathic medical college. In order to be licensed, we are then required to pass state or national board examinations, and our practices are subject to review by a state board of examiners.

The naturopathic medical student's first two years of college do not differ greatly from conventional medical school, as they include basic science courses and a study curriculum from standard medical textbooks. Our courses teach us how to use modern diagnostic and laboratory equipment, testing procedures, and how to administer prescription pharmaceuticals. But, it's our last two years of clinical training that set us apart from conventional doctors. During this time we learn the skills of a general family practitioner, just like our conventional medical counterparts, but with a distinctive guiding philosophy based on the following insights and principles. First, do no harm. Second, find the cause (just treating the symptoms is not enough). Third, use the healing power of nature. Fourth, treat the whole person. And fifth, use preventive medicine because the highest form of medicine is knowing how to stay healthy.

In practice, naturopathic physicians perform physical examinations and laboratory tests, and utilize X rays and other diagnostic procedures similar to a conventional doctor. We may also choose to perform nutritional, dietary, and digestive assessments, and inquire into the patient's mental and emotional well-being. And always, the patient is acknowledged as a participant in the healing process. Choosing a naturopathic physician does not mean disavowing conventional medicine. What it does mean is that you are choosing a doctor who understands and combines the best of what all forms of medicine have to offer. N.D.'s collaborate with all other branches of medicine, referring patients to appropriate specialists for their diagnosis or treatment whenever necessary. My practice has included gynecology, obstetrics, natural childbirth, pre- and postnatal care, pediatrics, sports medicine, and general family health, covering everything from allergies and cardiovascular health to diabetes and arthritis.

Given the dilemma most menopausal women face when choosing to take hormones, perhaps it isn't surprising that from the very beginning of my practice, the subject of menopause seemed to choose me. My patients' experiences taught me just how prevalent hormonal health problems are throughout a woman's life, and how often the current therapies not only offer less than a full treatment but come with myriad undesirable, uncomfortable, and downright deadly side effects. Tragically, even the women who experience relief without noticeable side effects still, and rightfully so, have grave health concerns. They don't want to give up feeling better on HRT, but they are desperately hoping that each checkup will not bring them a cancer diagnosis. The decisions these women are making are like a roll of the dice. They believe they have only two alternatives: HRT, weight gain, and the specter of cancer looming ever closer, or, facing the music of hot flashes, night sweats, mood swings, osteoporosis, heart disease, and the withering of youth.

My search for better, safer, and more effective ways to help my patients began in 1985 when one of my first truly challenging patients walked through my doors and changed my life forever. This patient's symptoms were multiple and very severe. She wanted relief as quickly as possible. She was hoping that I had an answer for her, and there was no way she would take a drug.

Originally my menopause protocol consisted of several herbal tinctures. Tinctures are made from herbs that have been steeped in alcohol for several weeks to extract their pharmacological and nutritional properties. I used herbs like angelica, dioscorea, motherwort, licorice, vitex, and ginseng, known to help a broad range of menopausal discomforts. Within days my patient felt better, within weeks she was feeling almost normal, and within the month she could actually wear a sweater, something she had been unable to do for quite some time because of her hot flashes and sweating. Her success led to dozens of immediate referrals. She sent a long list of friends and professional contacts to me.

Over time I found that the tinctures worked well, but that they had limitations. Most of them were bitter-tasting, they had to be taken frequently, they contained a high percentage of alcohol, it was inconvenient to carry the little bottles around, and they could cause the staining of tooth enamel. This inspired me to research effective hormone balancing and replenishing therapies and refine my protocol. I began using more capsules and tablets that contained herbs, herb concentrates, and nutritional components, and I relied less on the tinctures. Again, there was better than average success; however, the patients had to swallow a significant number of pills and the potency of the ingredients was variable, therefore the dosing had to be changed continually. These were great starts, but my patients and I needed more dependability, predictability, and convenience.

As natural therapies evolved, pharmaceutical standards were being applied to natural medicines. For example, natural remedies could now be purchased in standardized doses, just like most drugs. This meant that I could prescribe my protocols by using smaller doses and that my patients could take them more conveniently and less frequently. For my patients, that meant consistent dosing in an easy-to-take, recognizable form. Also, they could now choose whether they preferred using drops, capsules, suppositories, or skin creams as part of their programs. This improved my patients' responses significantly. My program today utilizes standardized extracts, concentrated herbal formulas, nutritional supplements, and plant-derived bio-identical hormones. With these advancements, my results have been effective and predictable.

In 1993, after having heard that I was treating women with

natural hormones, a new patient, Chris Conrad, came to see me. Following a complete hysterectomy, Chris had been suffering ill health with overlapping problems for four years. Her physical condition had deteriorated and her osteoporosis risk was severe, but Chris's gastrointestinal problems prevented her from continuing to take HRT drugs. Using a combination of plant-derived bioidentical hormone creams absorbed through the skin, plus rehabilitation for musculoskeletal loss of function with added digestive support for her malabsorption and other gastrointestinal problems, I was able to set Chris on the road to recovery. When she went back to her original doctors, they retested her. Chris's hormone levels had rebounded and were balanced, her osteoporosis risk was eliminated. In every way she was the best she had been in years. She was so relieved and happy that she wanted to share her good fortune with the world.

"No one I know has heard of this natural approach to menopause, and no one knows about these natural hormones," Chris told me. "Finding you was serendipity. You've got to write a book about this."

I was very busy with my practice, so I suggested that we collaborate, and the idea for *Natural Woman, Natural Menopause* was born.

Menopausal wellness is multifaceted. It is much more than just taking a pharmaceutical prescription, and far more than just estrogen replacement. It is not just the singular focus of one hormone, but is rather the interplay of all your hormones, which may, and often does, involve progesterone, testosterone, or DHEA, and their relationship to each other. Furthermore, osteoporosis prevention involves more than simply calcium supplementation, and may be more related to dietary magnesium, boron, and other minerals. It is absolutely essential in the building of strong bones that you have a balanced team of nutrients, trace elements, and exercise, all working together. And, even though prescription hormones can be part of your menopause program, it is important for you to know that all prescription hormones are not created equal. Knowing the differences can provide you with not only relief, but protection. If your doctor doesn't know which ones to prescribe, you need to know which ones to ask for.

We have lost touch with and have been seduced and advertised away from the potency and the effectiveness of our natural pharmacy. We have been led to believe that only pharmaceutical drugs have the power to cure our ills. This is far from the truth. In fact, it's the truth turned upside down. Synthetics can be powerful, but they always come with side effects. Many side effects are caused by your body's inability to recognize, utilize, or excrete concentrated alien substances. Natural substances come with natural buffering and synergistic agents that your body can use with ease. For example, raw honey, pure maple syrup, and real unrefined cane sugar (Sucanat) contain an array of beneficial minerals and nutrients, and these elements work as a team. Saccharin and cyclamates, synthetic sweeteners with no inherent health benefits, were originally approved as safe (not dissimilar to the way most promising new drugs enter the scene). A number of subsequent studies led to different conclusions. Cyclamates were removed from the marketplace in 1969 because they were found to cause cancer in laboratory animals, and saccharin has been implicated in many animal studies as causing precancerous lesions and cancer itself. These simple analogies offer insight into just a few of the differences between natural and synthetic remedies.

Research flooding the journals in the last few years is illuminating and identifying hundreds of healing agents in foods. These previously unknown phytochemicals are potent protectors, defenders, and promoters of your health. They occur naturally in commonly eaten fruits and vegetables, soybeans, whole grains, herbs, and spices. Many of them are part of a plant's own protection against its environment, and may provide you with the same kind of benefits—the prevention and treatment of disease. As our scientific understanding grows and the prejudice against nonpharmaceutical medicine erodes, the new research not only supports traditional healing practices, but offers proof of their potent efficacy. Medical science is now discovering what women's bodies have been telling them all along. Whether it is an antibiotic, a heart medication, a cancer treatment, or a hormone, nature provides a cure.

My experience and research have lead me to believe that what women have been told about their menopause and its treatment is neither accurate nor complete. The Natural Woman plan we are offering you today is the culmination of what worked in my practice, combined with the most current research. It is a streamlined, simple program for women and physicians to use—a natural lifestyle prescription that is hormonally healthy, cardiovascular-friendly, cancer resistant, and can make osteoporosis obsolete. It is a return to traditional wisdom. You can be sexually active, attractive, and vital throughout all of your years. Your menopause will be a liberating and rewarding transition into a positive, productive, and exciting rest of your life.

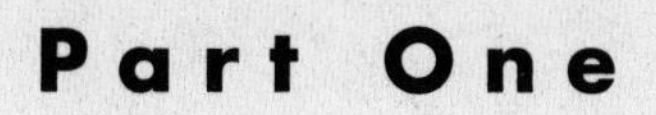
Part One

1

ANOTHER WAY

If you're an American woman over forty you'd have to be on Mars not to have heard at least *something* about "The Great Hormone Debate." To take or not to take hormone replacement therapy—this is the dilemma now faced by millions of women at menopause. Hormone replacement therapy (HRT) is the name given to a variety of estrogenic and synthetic progesterogenic products that are prescribed for menopausal symptoms, such as hot flashes and night sweats, and the prevention of osteoporosis and heart disease.

In the last five years the subject of menopause has been in the news more and more, as scores of magazine articles, books, and TV stories reel out scary scenarios that only contribute to a woman's confusion. On the one hand, there is the increasingly loud chorus of M.D.'s across the country extolling HRT's virtues and prescribing it for lifetime use.[1] On the other hand, many studies have pointed out the serious potential of uterine and breast cancer with long-term HRT use, not to mention the difficult and numerous side effects experienced by a sizable number of women who take these drugs.

A good part of what is driving the increasing attention to the subject of menopause is that contemporary women who have demanding lives and careers now see the years after forty as the full bloom of their productivity, and want to take control of the hormones in their bodies without feeling that there is something to be ashamed of.

If you're a woman who has begun to have hot flashes and experience the other bodily changes that signal the onset of menopause, you are thinking, Oh, God, it's happening to me, what do I do now? Do I just suffer through it? . . . The night sweats, the mood swings, the hot flashes, the dry and thinning skin . . . How long are these symptoms going to go on? Am I going to turn old overnight? Or do I take a chance with these drugs and live with the constant fear of getting cancer?

Maybe you've heard from one of your friends that she feels so much better taking her Premarin and Provera. Her mood has brightened, her skin looks better, and she has more energy. But then another friend told you she hated the stuff because the side effects were terrible and she gained twenty-five pounds! And you've heard of a woman taking Premarin for years who recently developed breast cancer.

It is definitely a head-splitting decision, which only compounds the fact that you have to deal with your roller-coaster emotions and, perhaps, the nagging nightly dream that you are turning into your mother.

But you can bypass all this agony—bypass playing Russian roulette with your health. There exists a genuinely safe, sensible, and effective way to balance and replenish your hormones. You can eliminate symptoms and protect your body while getting *all of the cosmetic benefits* but *none of the side effects and long-term risks of HRT.*

It's all true. "The Great Hormone Debate" is a fallacy. *There is another way* that is better, safer, and more effective. Approximately *two million U.S. women* are presently using with great success the products we will be recommending, and the number is expanding every day.[2] These women are part of a grassroots movement that is changing the "hormone" landscape for women in this country as one woman tells another, who then tells another. It is these pioneers who are demanding—and getting—better and safer treatment.

A Better Way

In this book, we will present you with a plan based on the following elements:

Replenishing of hormones using bio-identical plant-derived hormone products, which are plant extractions that exactly replicate your own hormones. These plant-derived hormones are almost entirely without the side effects of the synthetic or semisynthetic HRT drugs commonly prescribed. They can be prepared in an oral (pill), sublingual (under the tongue), cream, or gel form, and can be tailored to a woman's individual hormonal requirements.

These plant-derived hormones are now being prescribed by the full spectrum of health practitioners, including M.D.s, N.D.s, D.O.s (osteopaths), N.P.s (nurse practitioners), and other medical practitioners across the United States. Comparable products have been used effectively in Europe for over forty years.

They are available in FDA-regulated licensed pharmacies across the country. There is now a spreading network of *compounding* pharmacies that work with doctors to custom-design natural hormones for a woman's particular needs.

A specially designed eating plan for hormone balancing and replenishment. The foundations of this diet are scientifically, clinically, and epidemiologically supported, and based in part on the latest research and the findings of the exemplary Oxford-Cornell China diet study. It is foods from traditional diets that have now been shown to have beneficial effects throughout a woman's life in balancing hormonal levels.

An exercise plan based on the latest scientific research, which will keep you strong, fit, and toned, and can even help reverse any preexisting bone loss.

Supplementation with additional herbal products and nutrients to fortify you against the assaults on your system coming from pesticides, so-called *xenoestrogens,* and the stress of modern life, all of which can seriously unbalance your hormones without your being aware of it. (Xenoestrogens, also known as xenobiotics, are chemical substances in our environment that mimic human hormones and interfere with their functions. A further discussion of xenoestrogens will appear in subsequent chapters.)

Together, these elements of the Natural Woman plan, when adopted, can provide all the hormonal support a woman needs for the whole of her life.

But, you think, come on, what's the catch? Can I really get rid of my symptoms, have smoother skin, a glowing complexion, and a new, sexy attitude without taking my life in my hands, so to speak? Is there really an approach to menopause that is at once beneficial to my health, beautifying *and* medically safe, and even cancer-protective? Your M.D. internist/gynecologist may very well give you the impression that your choice is either Premarin, Ogen, another synthetic hormone, or nothing—or you must suffer through it. He/She may scare you into thinking you are doomed to heart disease and osteoporosis if you resist. At a recent symposium in Los Angeles, a well-known woman M.D. cancer specialist told the women in the audience, "There is no free lunch. If you want the benefits [of hormone therapy], you have to pay the price."[3] Well, that is true if you're taking Premarin, or synthetic hormones, but it doesn't have to be so.

Take, for example, Fay K. She had a complete hysterectomy at thirty-two. After ten years of taking the Premarin prescribed for her after the operation, she was plagued by weight gain, bloating, and gastrointestinal symptoms. After switching to a natural plant-derived estrogen/progesterone preparation, she lost twenty-five pounds in two months and her other symptoms disappeared.

Or Jane R., age fifty-four. Her doctor prescribed Premarin/Provera when her periods stopped. During the days she added Provera to her regimen, she reacted badly to it—it felt like the old days of PMS. Her doctor offered no other choice. Finally, a friend recommended replacing the Provera with natural progesterone *her* doctor had prescribed through a compounding pharmacy. Immediately, Jane no longer suffered her miserable symptoms. Months later, Jane, having educated herself on the overall superiority of "the naturals," switched from the Premarin to a plant-derived estrogen compound that the compounding pharmacy tailored to her needs. Now using both estrogen and progesterone in a natural form, she is completely symptom- and side-effect free.

Mary B., age forty-five. Despite the fact that she had a multitude of seemingly "menopausal" symptoms—including depression, agitation, sleeplessness, and hot flashes—Mary was told by her doctor that it was "too soon" for any kind of hormone replacement, as she was still menstruating and her estrogen levels were "normal." She was sent home with a prescription for an antidepressant and told to just live with the symptoms. She then went to Marcus Laux, who prescribed natural progesterone and a herbal product, Remifemin, which has been widely prescribed for hormonal complaints for more than forty years in Europe, and more recently in Australia and the U.S. She is now symptom-free and has never filled the prescription for the antidepressant.

Susan F., age forty-eight. Breast cancer runs in her family, and she was told by several doctors that she would therefore be unable to take hormone drugs for the hot flashes, night sweats, and other menopausal symptoms she was experiencing. Susan went to a new gynecologist, Uzzi Reiss, M.D., a Los Angeles doctor with a patient base of over 1,000 women using "the naturals," who was well versed in research from Europe and the United States that showed that *estriol,* a different estrogen from the one in the standard HRT, can actually be *cancer preventive.* Susan is now safely using natural plant-derived estriol (see chapter 8) along with natural progesterone for her menopausal symptoms.

Many women will be coming to this book already disillusioned with the way in which modern medicine treats women. Gail Sheehy's book *The Silent Passage* brought out into the open the dismal track record of physicians when it comes to menopause.[4] As she pointed out, gynecologists and internists by and large find the menopausal woman an unappealing patient. The vast majority of general practitioners are ill-informed on biological changes of women at midlife and are inclined to dismiss the symptoms as "psychological"—or if physiological effects are acknowledged, inconsequential. Women's health care is still in the Dark Ages in this country, and only recently is recognition being given to the problem. The director of a study initiated in 1995 by the National Institute on Aging is quoted in the *Los Angeles Times* as saying, "Women in this age period [40 to 55] have been understudied.

There is almost nothing [in medical literature] with respect to their physiology."[5] Medical models for disease are almost exclusively based on the masculine body and masculine experience. The unique hormonal changes that occur monthly in a woman do not get factored into the equation, for, in effect, modern medicine studies the anatomy of a woman's body as if it were simply a man's body with a reproductive system installed in it.[6] It is also a little known fact that almost all clinical drug trials use male subjects for their testing—even if the drug is targeted specifically for female use. This information surfaced recently when it was reported that the subjects in clinical trials for breast cancer drugs had all been men![7]

Putting Women at Risk Unnecessarily

Every day in the United States 3,500 women enter menopause. By the year 2000, there will be 50 million menopausal women in this country. It is estimated that 15 to 30 percent of the country's 40 million menopausal or post-menopausal women are on HRT synthetic hormones. *That's over 8 million women taking synthetic hormones today.*

The most common regimen prescribed by standard medical practitioners today is Premarin, a so-called conjugated estrogenic compound, combined with Provera, a synthetic progesterone derivative. In the late seventies, after studies showed that women taking Premarin alone were at risk for endometrial cancer, Provera was added as a protection for the endometrial lining. Women who have had their ovaries removed are generally only prescribed Premarin because it is believed that since they are not at risk for endometrial cancer, they don't need the protection of progesterone. Other common estrogenic drugs are Ogen and Orthoest, which though plant-derived are not identical to a woman's estrogen.

It has been estimated that as many as one-half of all women on the Premarin/Provera regime stop after a year, unable to tolerate the side effects. Two-thirds of all women stop the Provera (frequently without telling their doctors) and continue to take just Premarin, foregoing the more difficult side effects of Provera, which can mimic the worst of PMS symptoms, such as bloating, irritability, and depression. But by taking the Premarin alone they are putting themselves at potential risk for endometrial cancer.

And there are too many women who, because of the confusion and misinformation about HRT, forego any kind of help for hormonal imbalances and thereby end up suffering in silence.

It is hard to imagine a more serious situation for women in this country. A June 1995 *Time* magazine cover story described M.D.s as giving out "little red pills like M&Ms."[8] Despite claims by the pharmaceutical industry for the safety of the HRT drugs, *the eight million women presently on HRT are taking drugs that have been shown to have a significant health risk with long-term use.* The latest Nurses' Health Study, reported in *The New England Journal of Medicine*, which followed 121,700 women from 1978 to 1992, reported that women who take HRT for several years after menopause appear to raise their risk of breast cancer by nearly half.[9] Further testing of long-term usage of the Premarin/Provera regime continues, but the National Institutes of Health's Post-Menopausal Estrogen/Progesterone Intervention (PEPI) study will not be fully complete until 2005! Initial reports of the PEPI study have confirmed the benefits of using natural progesterone over Provera, although Provera still continues to be the choice of most standard practitioners. In the coming years, as the baby-boom generation enters menopause, the number of women at risk could rise dramatically.

The good news is that there are women who are trusting their instincts and refusing to take these prescription drugs. According to an article in the *Los Angeles Times* in 1994, "There's an enormous amount of resistance [to HRT] . . . In the last two years, physicians around the country have come to recognize that many women have dug in their heels about this. Doctors are wondering what they can do differently to get women to take it."[10]

Many of these resistant women are saying to themselves: *Wait a minute. Something's not right here. How can it be that the best thing for my health after fifty is to take a prescription drug with known cancer risks for the rest of my life? This can't be my only choice.*

And perhaps some of these women have long memories—remembering other drugs, like DES or thalidomide, which were at first touted as safe but later turned out to have tragic health consequences in the children of the mothers who used them.

Feeling Safe

The onset of menopause can strike fear in a woman's heart. Suddenly a body you once thought you knew well starts to "misbehave"—you experience temperature changes, hot sweats, cold sweats, weight gain, mood swings, and a lack of concentration. Or possibly your skin is changing, you get urinary tract infections, and intercourse is suddenly painful. What's going on here, who is this woman?

This is not a time when you want to go sailing out into unknown territory. You want to do something positive for yourself, but you also want to feel that what you're doing is safe, sensible, and effective. You certainly don't want to risk cancer for the purported cosmetic benefits of HRT.

In *The Silent Passage,* Gail Sheehy was the first mainstream writer to talk about the value of the natural plant-derived hormones, in particular, natural progesterone, and she encouraged women to seek out natural remedies. She herself had little knowledge of them and told readers to be prepared to spend *a year* experimenting because of the wide variety of herbal possibilities.[11]

If you're a woman who took this advice and went about looking for answers in books on a natural approach to menopause, you probably ended up very frustrated. First, you would find many books that advertised themselves as "natural," but were, in fact, anything but. Many interesting and useful books that advocate natural remedies are available, but the dizzying lists of herbal remedies tied to specific symptoms can overwhelm the reader with too many different and sometimes conflicting remedies, many with exotic names unfamiliar to us as children of Western medicine—names such as dong quai, vitex agnus castus, horsetail, evening primrose oil, and so on. We're sure you're already busy enough without having to become an amateur chemist or herbalist. How many women have the time or expertise to make herbal tinctures? Excepting the dedicated few, what most women end up with is a fistful of receipts, a shelfful of bottles of expensive *stuff,* and just more uncertainty and confusion.

The Best of Both Worlds

What *Natural Woman* provides is a combination of the best in Western scientific methods and analysis with natural healing principles that are supported by thousands of years of herbal knowledge. The world of natural medicine may have once seemed suspiciously "New Age" to Americans, but there is now a quiet and steady revolution occurring as more and more people in this country are showing an interest in using natural substances for healing. Women coming into menopause today are among that growing segment of the the U.S. population paying more visits to "alternative practitioners" than to all "conventional" doctors combined (according to a study published in 1990 in *The New England Journal of Medicine*). Most likely, someone you know is now using *echinacea* combined with *goldenseal* for his or her cold symptoms and swears by it. *Ginkgo biloba,* an herb used for centuries to improve circulation, has been the number-one-selling prescription drug in Germany and France and is gaining popularity in the United States. "Consumers are becoming aware of the restrictive nature of U.S. drug-approval policies and are increasingly comfortable relying upon medical findings from other scientifically advanced countries . . . The broad acceptance of herbs in Europe has finally captured the attention of Americans . . ." says an article in the *Los Angeles Times* in November 1995.[12]

Nothing attests to the growing importance of natural medicine in the United States more than the fact that insurance companies are beginning to pay for natural medicine regimes. The Oxford Health Plan of Connecticut has added an alternative medicine program and has recruited 1,000 alternative care practitioners including naturopaths as primary care doctors for this HMO. The first state-funded natural medicine clinic, King County Natural Medicine, has recently opened in Washington State, and, spurred by popular demand, a Congressionally mandated office for alternative medicine was recently established by the National Institutes of Health. And there is now a growing number of M.D.s who, for menopausal care, are breaking away from the synthetic hormone regime and have joined naturopaths, acupuncturists, and other holistic practitioners in prescribing plant-derived hormones along with dietary changes.

Why? Because they find that it works. Patients are satisfied.

Their physicians can prescribe the plant-derived hormones in standardized doses specifically tailored to their individual midlife profiles, For many conventional practitioners, it is a difficult but rewarding learning curve, moving them from outside the sphere of influence of "medicine by advertising." Many doctors have been led to believe that almost all products are interchangeable, or that a particular treatment can work for everyone. Not true. Doctors like Andrew Weil and Deepak Chopra have done a great deal in promoting the popular understanding of the body as an interacting complexity, and have demonstrated the benefits of harnessing the wisdom of thousands of years of plant medicine. But, ultimately, practitioners trained in mainstream medical schools are moving in this direction *because their patients are demanding it.*

The Natural Woman Solution

We will provide you with complete information about the use of bio-identical plant-derived hormones—which we believe are better, safer, and more effective than synthetic drugs. The natural estrogen and progesterone products derived from plants *match your own hormones exactly*, something that cannot be said of Premarin and Provera, the two most heavily prescribed drugs for menopause.

You will learn how menopause has been "medicalized," or turned from a natural passage into a disease that then needs to be treated with HRT drugs. Much of the confusion surrounding HRT comes from accepting without question the presumptions of our present medical system.

Balance

You will learn about natural hormone replenishment and balancing, and how the principle of *balance* is fundamental to a smooth passage through menopause. The so-called *sex hormones*—e.g., estrogen, progesterone, testosterone—are, in fact, all created from the same source (cholesterol) and work in the body in a kind of symphonic blending, *morphing* from each other and *depending* on each other. No hormone in the body works in isolation. The brain, the endocrine system, and the immune system are not separate entities, but partners working in a close relationship, which is one reason the view of menopause as an estrogen-deficiency disease is dangerously narrow. Keeping your hormones balanced is the key to well-being.

Progesterone, the Neglected Hormone

In the emphasis on replacing estrogen in the body, the importance of the hormone *progesterone* to the midlife woman has been overlooked. The very latest studies of how progesterone works in the body indicate that it has very important functions beyond ovulation in the female. According to these recent studies, progesterone is at least as important as estrogen in the prevention of osteoporosis—it can actually *build* new bone, which most estrogenic products cannot.[13] And according to a 1995 *New York Times* article, French researchers reported that progesterone may play a "previously unrecognized role" in helping to repair and replace the protective covering around nerves,[14] which suggests that this hormone has many unrecognized values for a woman after midlife. And in the most important study of progesterone to date, this "neglected" hormone has been shown to play a potentially important role in the protection of breast tissue from cancer[15] and the protection of coronary arteries against vasospasm. You will learn about the importance of supplementing estrogen *and* progesterone, not estrogen alone, for the hysterectomized woman—a serious omission in standard medical treatment, which will be discussed further in chapters 9 and 10.

Testosterone and DHEA

More and more information is surfacing on how these critically important but less understood *androgen* hormones have a significant impact on a woman's midlife health, and how they can be used to your benefit. Androgen refers to those hormones, produced in both men and women, known to promote, among various functions, masculine characteristics. Although the amount of testosterone in a woman's body is much lower than in a man's, it is equally important to a woman's well-being. Testosterone has important functions in the female body in maintaining sexual vitality, general energy, and in actually *building* bone and maintaining muscle.[16] The ratio of testosterone to estrogen and progesterone is also vital to preventing unwanted body changes, such as weight gain, at midlife. And for the woman who has had a hysterectomy, replacement can be a necessity.

Until recently, little was known about DHEA, a *precursor* hormone from which other sex hormones are made. But the very latest studies show how this hormone may have important therapeutic effects for many medical problems, including cardiovascular disease, Alzheimer's disease, and osteoporosis.

Diet

You will learn how diet is fundamental to navigating the menopausal passage. In Japan, where there isn't a word for "hot flashes" in the language, women have a diet heavily dependent on vegetable and soy products, such as tofu, which contain potent phytohormones. Studies have shown that when these women change to a Western diet, they begin to experience the common symptoms of menopause. In cases where women have resumed the traditional diet, it's been shown that their menopausal symptoms again disappear.[17] Despite this clear link between diet and menopausal symptoms, it is the rare American physician who will even ask you about your dietary habits.

And not only is this diet good for menopause, it is good for your overall health as well, as general health has a major effect on how your body handles menopause, another important issue rarely recognized in the general practitioner's office. The diet we have designed is supported by the newest understanding of phytonutrients and "nutraceuticals"—natural substances in food that have physiologic action and are not classified as drugs—and is further supported by the leading study on diet and disease, the Oxford-Cornell China diet study. You will get the benefit of all the new scientific understanding of "food as medicine."

In addition, you will learn about the important link between *hormone balancing and digestion,* something you are unlikely to hear about in the standard practitioner's office. Just as digestive functioning is crucial to the management of your overall health, so it is to your "hormonal health." If you're absorbing nutrients poorly, then you may not be properly absorbing the estrogen or progesterone you are taking for replenishment. We will guide you in the proper use of "probiotics," those "good" bacteria that help you absorb nutrients properly and which are necessary to help maintain hormonal balance.

Supplementation

You will learn what supplementation of essential vitamins and nutrients you need to take to fight off the stresses of the environment. Our polluted environment and the pressures of modern life tax your hormonal system and can accelerate menopausal symptoms. Finding the right supplementation can be intimidating and confusing, with endless choices and varieties being touted as the answer. We'll set the record straight and give you a plan that will strengthen and build vitality.

Exercise

We will tell you what exercise is best for you. Couch potatoes, prepare yourselves—exercise is not optional. A certain amount of weight-bearing exercise is mandatory for the health of your bones, to eliminate the possibility of osteoporosis in your life. We need to look at exercise as a *component* of health, not an option, not something that just helps us get rid of flabby thighs. Studies have shown that exercise is a factor in the prevention of breast cancer,[18] and it is also a factor in the balancing of the hormones in your body.

Care of the Skin

Your face and body can be the splendid beneficiaries of a new generation of products that take advantage of the hormonal actions of plant extractions and fruit acids—no small matter to a woman who wants to look vital and rejuvenated. Creams with a progesterone or estriol content, or with essential oils from plants and plant juices, prevent free-radical damage, slough off dead skin, and plump up and rejuvenate the skin.

We have divided the book into two parts. Part One sets out to untangle the present confusion over HRT, in addition to providing a grounding in natural medicine for those who are completely unfamiliar with it, and a scientific rationale for the use of plant-derived hormones and how they work. The book is designed so that each chapter leads you one step closer to making an informed decision. We urge all women and practitioners who work with women to make themselves familiar with these issues, as they can have important implications for overall health as well.

For those who want immediate access to the practical recommendations or feel they already have the necessary grounding in the issues, you can skip to Part Two and refer back to Part One as a reference.

Better Than Ever

It may be hard to believe, but menopause is a genuine opportunity to re-create yourself: It is the ultimate "wake-up call," telling you to pay attention to your health and prepare yourself for the second part of your life. To pass through your menopause naturally does not mean fatalistically accepting whatever hormonal withering comes over you. Menopause, as with all life's transitions, is not an ending but an awakening.

In many cultures, the cessation of menstruation is often cause for celebration. In these cultures, a woman is given *more* freedom and *more* status and is revered for her wisdom and her social and political skills. Freed from the constraints of child-rearing, women can take positions as civic leaders and contribute to the well-being of their people. In the Kung society of Africa, the older women took on young lovers and became the revered teachers of sexuality to the young.[19] Women in our society—principally the baby boomers, who have become accustomed to positions of power in the workplace—should be heartened by the fact that there is ample precedent for a lusty and powerful second part of life. Unfortunately, everything in American culture works against a woman facing the end of menstruation: the constant emphasis on looking young and the lack of respect for old age, and the strong subliminal belief that life is a constant upward movement toward success, never allowing for the *end* of anything.

Denial

If you live in a society that stigmatizes "The Change," the last thing you want to do is admit to yourself or anyone else that it's happening to you. It can seem to many women a cruel joke that their body starts to go haywire just when they have come to feel that they are at the top of their game.

Letting a spouse in on it can compound the trauma. Many women fear that their husbands will no longer find them sexually attractive once the word "menopause" enters the bedroom. After all, he may be struggling with his own midlife change, and he's a child of American culture as well.

And there is the definite sadness that can come—particularly if you loved being a mother and raising your children—of knowing that your child-bearing years are over. Or if you're not married, or never had children, then you might be overcome with a sense of life having passed you by.

But denial can be your worst enemy. It can keep you from getting help with unwanted symptoms, keep you in a cycle of needless discomfort, and even jeopardize your future health. Initial denial is probably inevitable in every woman, but the sooner a woman gets over the denial hump the better.

Because there is every reason to take heart. The stereotypes of old women rendered useless and sent out to pasture are just that, *stereotypes.* You can come through this passage reawakened, with a greater feeling of wellness, of energy, of sexual attractiveness, renewed for the coming best years of your life.

But we are going to ask you to do no less than suspend any of your prejudices as best you can, and to realize that you may have to *revolutionize* your thinking and get into a totally different mindset.

To our knowledge, there is no other book available that provides a complete plan for a healthy menopause. If you're anticipating menopause, are in menopause, or are maintaining your health post-menopause, this is the book for you. We give you a basic blueprint, which will work for most women, with advice on how to adjust it for your specific needs. If you follow our plan, we'll save you much of the trial and error.

We think this is the optimum plan for most women to follow,

as it is based on the latest scientific research and backed up by much of the very research that is being prepared by drug companies.

The overwhelming emotion coming over a woman in menopause is loss of control of her body. We want to give you the knowledge that you can take hold of your biochemistry and come out of the passage mentally and physically stronger, and even *more beautiful*—in every way more powerful than when you began. Give us and yourself six months' time.

2

"ESTROGEN": THE MISUNDERSTOOD HORMONE

From the very day it enters a woman's mind that replacing hormones is something she should think about, she will immediately enter a zone of conflicting information and loose facts and prejudices from the media, her friends, her internist, her gynecologist, or her mother, all mixing together with her own preexisting ideas into a confusing stew. So before we can even *begin* to discuss our plan, we need to clear away some misunderstandings and misinformation.

"*Taking estrogen is dangerous.*" How many women have you heard say this? If we could single out the most damaging consequence of the controversy over HRT, it would be that *estrogen*—this essential life-enhancing friend to your body—has become for many women a dirty word.

What Is "Estrogen"?

Since the first hormone replacement drugs were put on the market over fifty years ago, it has become an ingrained practice to use the word "estrogen" indiscriminately for both the estrogen your body produces and a wide range of diverse hormonal preparations. Drug companies with hormone replacement products have contributed significantly to the confusion by continually referring to their products as simply "estrogen."

A woman will tell a friend that she is taking estrogen, thinking she is ingesting a single substance called estrogen that conforms to the hormone produced in her own body. But estrogen is, in fact, not a *single* hormone but a *family* of hormones, consisting principally of estrone (E1), estradiol (E2), and estriol (E3). Along with these three principal estrogens, we know that there are at least *two dozen*[1] identified estrogens produced in a woman's body, and researchers may well discover others. Premarin contains 48 percent estrone (natural to humans) and 52 percent horse estrogens (natural to horses). It also contains additives that are foreign to a woman's body. None of the American drug products contain estriol (E3), which has been used widely in Europe for over fifty years, and which new studies have shown to be cancer preventive.[2] Estriol, the estrogen most dominant during pregnancy, has particular benefit for women who are at risk for breast cancer and need hormone balancing and replenishment. In Europe, it is particularly favored for use in vaginal preparations, such as Oevestin. The reasons for its being completely ignored in the United States until recently will be discussed at greater length in chapter 6.

Most media reporting contributes to the confusion over "estrogen" by failing to make clear which estrogen they are referring to or to make distinctions as to what specific products are being discussed or tested. None of the mainstream media articles reporting the recent studies of increased incidence of breast cancer in women on HRT mentioned the fact that the subjects had used Premarin. Of the three principal estrogens circulating in a woman's body, the one predominantly implicated in increased cancer risk is *estradiol.* Premarin, as noted, is formulated with estrone, which converts to estradiol. Estriol, as we have just mentioned, has *cancer-preventive* properties. So when the results of studies are announced that show increased risk of breast cancer in those women on HRT, it is unfortunately *estrogen* that is demonized and not the specific products tested.

The fact is, you cannot live without estrogen. Estrogen is not merely a "sex" hormone, as there are presently *three hundred known functions* for estrogen in the body and we are only beginning to understand all its interactions. Every cell in your body has *receptors*—what you might think of as little landing docks—that receive the complex hormonal messages circulating through your blood. There are estrogen receptors in all your vital organs—such as your brain, your heart, and your liver—and all through your body. Estrogen spurs the production of an important enzyme in the brain that helps the connections between brain cells to flourish. It is estrogen that helps maintain verbal learning and enhances a woman's capacity for new learning.[3] Indeed, estrogen supports you from birth until death.

Ironically, most of the studies relating to HRT products have gone very far to show what an important role your own naturally produced estrogen plays in the functioning of your body. But in its rush to give women the benefits of estrogen, the medical/pharmaceutical establishment has simply continued to promote the standard hormone products now available from the major drug companies without looking for better and safer alternatives that also don't have the negative side effects of the standard drugs.

Does "Estrogen" Cause Cancer?

Almost all the studies that link estrogen to an increased risk of cancer have been related to taking Premarin or other common drug products. Premarin is extracted from horse urine. While it contains helpful estrogens like *estrone* and *estradiol*, it also contains *equilin and equilenin* (horse estrogens) and synthetic additives. It is the taking of unbalanced and foreign estrogenic elements and additives that we believe is dangerous and potentially cancer producing, not estrogen itself. When used appropriately, the estrogen from natural plant sources, which matches your own hormones exactly, does not produce harmful side effects.

Standard medical practice prescribes drugs using the so-called risk/benefit factor. The side effects of a drug are medically accepted hazards of treatment: The judgment is made that the benefits outweigh the risks, and doctors are willing to accept the fact that you may suffer serious consequences. But are *you* willing to accept it?

A major link between raised estrogen levels and breast cancer is primarily a ratio problem—the ratio between estrogen and progesterone in your body, which can be brought on by poor diet, poor digestion, lifestyle habits, stress, or environmental factors. In the simplest terms, unbalanced estrogen-to-progesterone levels can cause a relative or absolute "estrogen dominance," which can lead to the proliferation of cancer cells. When the first hormone replacement drugs were put on the market, the symptoms of menopause were understood primarily in terms of "estrogen deficiency," but this has since proved to be a narrow vision. This erroneous medical model takes one hormone, *estrogen,* out of context in the body's functioning, and neglects the importance of *progesterone.* Just by correcting diet and digestion, you can decrease your environmental exposure and improve your body's ability to balance estrogen and progesterone and eliminate estrogen dominance. A plant-rich diet helps eliminate estrogen dominance and is actively anticarcinogenic.

But I Love My Premarin

On the other side of the aisle from those women who have an undifferentiated fear of estrogen are those women who simply continue to take Premarin or Premarin/Provera or the other commonly prescribed HRT drugs and shut their ears to all controversy.

Let us say right up front that we are not against "hormone replacement" per se, although what we are advocating could more accurately be called hormone *balancing* or *replenishment.* When it comes to dealing with temporary symptoms, such as hot flashes, night sweats, and vaginal dryness, Premarin has been shown to be effective. But we do think it is a crude product—crude in the sense that it was developed during the early stages of hormone investigation and contains estrogens foreign to a woman's body. We think this lack of conformity to a woman's body is what contributes to its side effects.

Those women who are able to tolerate Premarin can go on taking it for years—well past the five-year mark that most studies consider a critical period—all the while harboring the worry that if they go off it, the chassis will start to break down and various parts will begin to fail or fall off. These women face a difficult dilemma: If the drug they are using seems to be working, it's hard to consider a change. But ignoring the potential for harm can be dangerous to your health.

To add another complication, Premarin and its sister drugs are now being advertised as necessary to ward off osteoporosis and heart disease, opening up a whole new marketing strategy to sell these drugs to you for long-term use. When they were first put on the market, the primary emphasis was on short-term treatment of temporary symptoms, but by advocating use of these drugs for long-term use as prevention against heart disease and osteoporosis, a whole new element of danger and confusion has been added.

The Profit Motive

Why haven't the makers of standard HRT drugs sought out safer alternatives? In the case of Premarin, 940 million dollars and growing is the answer. Premarin is the number-one best-selling drug in the country.[4] Why haven't American pharmaceutical companies strongly marketed these safer bio-identical plant-derived hormone products? Simple. They can't be patented, which means that no single company can corner the market. And since research money will flow only to those projects that will provide a drug company with so-called *protected* profit, "natural" will almost always lose to "synthetic" in the pharmaceutical world.

If, for example, a pharmaceutical company decides to market a natural substance, another competing company could ride on its coattails and dilute its profitability, hence the notion of creating drugs with *protected* profit. Many natural substances are changed into patentable drugs simply by changing a few molecules of the natural substance. The decision to do this is often not driven by the desire for a better drug, but rather for one that is different enough to obtain a patent.

But what seems a *tiny* change in the molecular structure of a substance can make a huge difference in its effect on your body. Adding or subtracting a few hydrogen atoms and a few double bonds in the biochemical structure of estrogen or testosterone is the difference between a male and a female! In the case of Provera, which is a molecularly altered version of natural progesterone, side effects can result because the body doesn't recognize the substance as completely biologically identical to one in your body.

Fortunately, switching to the plant-derived bio-identical hormones can be done with relative ease. A woman taking Premarin can have an equivalent dose worked out for her by a pharmacist, and she can immediately start taking the plant-derived hormones.

How "Estrogen" Got Politicized

Unfortunately, and for many of the wrong reasons, *not* supplementing estrogen has become a political cause for some women.

Betty Friedan has taken a strong position against women using HRT. She is also quoted as saying, "I may have had a hot flash, *one* hot flash, while I was giving a major speech in the middle of the seventies,"[5] implying that women who took *anything* for menopause were sissies, and dismissing the significance of the menopausal passage altogether.

Well, Friedan is one lucky woman if she only had one hot flash she can barely remember. It probably means she has naturally favorable hormone levels either because of good genetics or her diet, and she is apparently among the 25 percent of women who sail through menopause without symptoms.

But what about the other 75 percent? These women are not as fortunate. Whether because of a complete hysterectomy, or just having their ovaries removed, less favorable genetics, a poor diet, or high stress levels—just to mention a few of the possibilities—these women can become noticeably and often severely symptomatic.

One third of women in this country have had hysterectomies (a shocking number, which we will talk about in a later chapter), and *all* of these women have suffered a hormonal "disruption" of some magnitude and will need help in replacing and balancing.

The impulse to shield women from drugs that are potentially harmful is a good one, but unfortunately, estrogen itself has become demonized rather than the specific products that have been shown to pose risks for a woman's health.

The negative result is that women who would benefit greatly

from the right kind of hormone replenishment or from a treatment plan that would help them deal with uncomfortable symptoms during menopause don't reach out and get the help they deserve.

Turning a Blind Eye to Menopause

Some women choose to deny the existence of menopause altogether, as if acknowledging it would be admitting that there is a difference between men and women. And some women have even gone so far as to insist that the studying of masculine and feminine differences is subversive to the feminist cause.

From a medical point of view, denying the difference between the sexes can actually have very serious negative consequences and can compound an existing problem. If, as we've said, medical treatment in the United States today is fundamentally based on a male body, then from a diagnostic point of view women are *already* treated like men—but very *unequal* men. The problems that are unique to women—in this case, hormonal fluctuations and imbalances—have historically been ignored or have been treated as emotional problems. In fact, the word "hysterical" comes from the Greek word for uterus. In the nineteenth century, the typical English doctor would simply remove the uterus when a woman displayed what to his mind was excessive emotionality. The medical literature is dismayingly rife with such examples. To deny the physical uniqueness of a woman is to collude with the prejudice that women have irritatingly aberrant male bodies.

The debate about hormones is being carried on in the wrong arena. The question is not *if* you should take hormone replacement therapy drugs, but *what* constitutes a healthy and vital body at menopause and *what* specific actions and products you should use to manage symptoms and restore balance to support your hormonal system.

What Is "Unnatural"?

Some women decide that they will just let menopause run its course, because taking supplements for it isn't *natural.* But the fact is that contemporary life for women has become very *unnatural.* Over hundreds of thousands of years of evolution, humans have developed sustaining behaviors for their strength and longevity, such as eating a plant-rich diet and moving their muscles regularly. But in the short span of perhaps fifty years, processed foods and preservatives and a more and more sedentary lifestyle have virtually eliminated many of these body-sustaining behaviors from our lives.

It's not *natural* to eat processed food.

It's not *natural* to eat anything synthetic that doesn't exist in nature.

It's not *natural* to forego the important foods that can help balance your hormones.

It's not *natural* to go without physical exercise.

It's not *natural* to live in a polluted environment.

Almost all this "unnaturalness" is imposed from *without*—from the polluted environment, the stress of maintaining two-income households, eating processed food for convenience, or getting less exercise due to labor-saving devices. But these factors have a negative impact on a woman's hormonal balance and overall health, and may ultimately be linked to her seemingly "sudden" menopausal symptoms and "sudden" ill health.

The underlying impulse to stay "natural" is a good one, but women who are saying this may not be thinking the issue through. How far would you be willing to take the "It's not natural" idea? Does this mean saying no to lotion for dry skin? No to lubrication for sexual comfort? No to vitamins? Staying "natural" need not mean rejecting the use of beneficial and safe products to counteract the toxicity of our environment and food supply and help balance hormonal function.

Many of the women who resist the idea of taking *anything* at menopause don't realize that at the same time they may be unquestioningly taking a variety of prescription drugs, such as the acid blockers Zantac and Tagamet, which are potentially harmful and hardly natural.

If saying "I'm not going to do anything for menopause, it's not natural" is just providing yourself with an excuse to stop taking care of yourself, well, unfortunately, there's nothing we can do to stop you. But acceptance of a normal and important passage of your life is not the same thing as giving in to aging—that is, allowing yourself to slowly balloon out, forget about sexuality, and then eventually sit down for good.

There are women who believe that God meant us to have low hormonal levels after a certain age, so that's how it should be. But think about this: Many Japanese women on their traditional diet have phytoestrogen levels in their urine that are *1,000 times higher* than those of U.S. women. This high excretion level means that their diet is so rich in beneficial plant food that all during their lives they have been "supplementing" their hormones naturally. When these women reach menopausal age, they don't have the symptoms so common to Western women. And if this were not reason enough to follow such a diet, *these women rarely get breast cancer.*[6]

The plants are much smarter than the man-made synthetics. They help you to up-regulate and down-regulate your hormone levels naturally. Unlike Premarin, which contains estrogens that are foreign to your body, and which may slow down the process of excretion, the plant substances are excreted very quickly. This is important because the longer an estrogen foriegn to humans stays in the body, the more opportunity it has to cause you problems in the form of side effects.

Our need for hormones continues through our lifetimes. So yes, menstruation will cease, yes, your ovaries will no longer be producing estrogen and progesterone the way they used to—*but hormones will still play a very important part in maintaining your bodily functions.* And keeping their levels appropriate and balanced with diet and supplementation will support you healthfully and vitally through old age.

But Grandma Never Took Hormones . . .

Women concerned about whether hormone replacement is "natural" often argue that previous generations seemed to have gotten along fine without it. This is a very good point, and again speaks to the confusion created by the drug industry and the medical establishment. Pharmaceutical companies have worked hard to induce a fear state in which women begin to think their bones will turn to dust and their hearts will stop working if they don't take their prescription drugs for the rest of their lives.

These claims are indeed worthy of a good deal of skepticism, especially if the drugs come with significant expense, side effects, and cancer risks.

However, there is still good reason for you to pay attention to your "hormonal health" by balancing and replenishing with plant-derived hormones. Why? Because you and your grandmother may be different in very important ways.

First, we don't really know the exact state of your grandmother's health. Just how healthy is she? Just how active is she? How does she look for her age? And given the reticence of previous generations on matters pertaining to their bodies, it would be hard to know what she may or may not have suffered during menopause. "The Change" has only recently become a topic of public or even private conversation. Also, we don't know what her diet consisted of. If she ate a healthy, preservative-free diet concentrated on fresh vegetables and fruits, then she got a plant-hormone-rich infusion all her life and didn't need to supplement. If she was active and worked her body regularly, then she got enough exercise to keep her bones strong and healthy.

But now we're talking about *you,* her granddaughter. If you've lived on processed foods and your dietary habits run to Häagen-Daz, coffee, and hamburgers on the run, if you don't move that body of yours but instead spend most of your day behind a desk, if you're supermom juggling a career and family, if you diet incessantly, yo-yoing up and down, if you've taken lots of antibiotics and prescription drugs, then you can't compare yourself with your grandmother. Genetics is only one factor, and may not be the biggest influence. Sure, if you and your grandmother are both lucky genetically, then she may have sailed through menopause and so might you, but there is no guarantee that this will happen to you. A whole different set of contemporary factors comes into play. For starters, your grandmother didn't have to fight off the onslaught of the pollutants of our present environment. She did not grow up on a diet of commercially grown food lacking in nutrients—especially essential minerals—and, unfortunately, very rich in pesticide residue, drugs, and chemical contaminants. And no previous generation has faced today's unique stress levels.

But this does not mean that your body is not *biologically* and *genetically* prepared to live to a ripe old age.

Living Longer . . . and Better

An insidious idea has taken hold in the menopause literature: We are told that because women are living longer than ever before (supposedly without precedent in human history), a woman's body after fifty is, so to speak, hormonally unprepared to live very much longer and cannot protect itself against the ravages of old age. This idea has been embraced by the medical profession to justify putting women on permanent HRT beginning at age fifty.

In previous centuries, the mean age of death for women may have been very low as women died as infants, as young children, in childbirth, as victims of epidemics, in famines, in war, etc., but this does not mean that these women were not *biologically* prepared to live very long lives. Medical anthropologist Margaret Lock, writing in *Lancet* in 1990, said: "Since there is evidence that people have lived to a very old age for at least 100,000 years, this means that from an *evolutionary* point of view the female body is biologically prepared to do so. The maximum life span *potential* for a woman is estimated to be about 92 years."[7] (The authors add: "We feel even this is short—and not the actual longevity potential. To prove our point, the oldest known person living today is a 120-year-old woman residing in France."[8])

In the early fifties, certain doctors began to define menopause as a disease—"estrogen deficiency" disease—which then needed to be treated with a drug. Traditional Asian medicine—which, by the way, is based on a "clinical trial" of at least a 2,000-year heritage and 400 unbroken generations of *written* patient experience—views menopause in an entirely different way than does standard medical practice in the United States. To the Asians, menopause is a necessary and vital process for the body's health. While obviously a signal that the woman has reached a certain age, passing through menopause actually serves to slow down the aging process by preventing the unnecessary loss of blood and *jing,* or essence, thus allowing the woman the possibility of good health for at least the next thirty years of life. To ensure a smooth passage in this "second spring" of a woman's life, Chinese doctors will prescribe tonics and other herbal remedies to balance the woman's hormones.[9] For thousands of years, Chinese women could live to a healthy old age—and what's more, they were venerated for it!

Looking Younger Than Ever

What has become evident in the United States is that women act and look *younger* for their age than in previous generations—forty today is what thirty was twenty years ago. Actresses can now actually be sexy onscreen past forty—Susan Sarandon, Jessica Lange, and Meryl Streep, to name just a few—which was not true a generation ago. Marilyn Monroe was considered over the hill at thirty-six. And now fifty for a woman is what forty was twenty years ago.

What's the secret? One thing we know is that these contemporary actresses are taking very good care of themselves. In fact, American women in general are taking advantage of a physical youthfulness that has been biologically possible for a long time. And they don't want to sink into the "Age fifty plus spends her life in the doctor's office" syndrome.

We're on the side of looking good at any age. We believe there is such a thing as healthy vanity. Wanting to look and feel beautiful is a woman's right. Some women have defensively embraced the idea of an old age *with* wrinkles and *without* sex. That's certainly an option. But any expectation you may have that after fifty you will turn into an old woman sitting on a park bench talking about her ailments is the function of an *acculturated* image. It doesn't have to be that way.

But the first step in taking full charge of your "second spring" is getting on good terms with your hormones—that is, understanding how they work in your body, and what you need to do to keep them balanced—and most important, learning how the plant-based diets and herbal medicines have supported human life for millions of years and are crucial to the well-being of women.

3

THE POWER OF PLANT HORMONES

When told that it's possible to synthesize hormones from plants that exactly match human hormones, most people will react with surprise. They are even more surprised to hear that plants themselves have their own hormonal systems. To appreciate the validity and superiority of using the plant-derived hormone preparations, it is important to understand the overall value that plants have for your well-being.

Millions of years before humans appeared on this planet, there were plants. In order to survive into the present, these plants became master biochemists, producing sophisticated chemical agents for their own protection and healing. In the wild and in your home, a plant manufactures "phytochemicals" to protect itself from threats to its survival such as life-giving yet potentially harmful sunlight, viruses, bacteria, and predators like insects.

Plants have their own version of an endocrine system just as you do. They produce a form of hormones, the "chemical messengers" that direct operations in their systems and have their own form of estrogenic and progesteronic substances just like yours.

You may think that the ficus plant sitting over there in a corner of your room leads a dull life, that it's just decoration, just sitting there waiting to be watered by you. But while this plant is sitting there in the corner, it is also:

Breathing. A million or so moving "lips" are sucking in carbon dioxide and expelling oxygen.

Moving. Though rooted, a plant can move its body freely, easily, and gracefully, and the only reason we don't appreciate this fact is because plants do so at a much slower rate than do humans.

Drinking. With its roots working as a water pump, moisture is constantly rising from root to leaf.

Seeking out light. The turn of the century botanist Raoul France demonstrated that plants are capable of *intent.* They *stretch* toward and *seek* out light just as a human would.

Protecting. A plant seems to know when a thief is in its territory and will shut down its nectar source when threatened.

Hearing. Plants have been found to be able to distinguish between sounds inaudible to the human ear and color wavelengths such as infrared and ultraviolet, invisible to the human eye.

Communicating. It is an accepted botanic principle that plants can *feel,* and can respond to human communication.

And, of course: *Growing.* A plant's endocrine system regulates this process. It may not have a menstrual cycle, but otherwise its hormones regulate growth and maturation in a process comparable in concept to yours.

In fact, plants possess and fulfill all the attributes of living creatures. According to *The Secret Life of Plants,* by Peter Tompkins and Christopher Bird, there is an abundance of evidence that now supports the thesis that plants are living, breathing, communicating creatures endowed with personality and attributes of the soul.[1]

Plants and Humans: An Enduring Connection

When we consume plants, they, in effect, pass on their chemical powers to us. *We are dependent on plants for our survival.* It is not simply that we need them for their "food" value—for proteins, fats, carbohydrates, etc.—but also for their *strategies* for survival, for their phytochemical arsenal. This is why "eat your vegetables" has been important advice since time immemorial.

Of the 375 billion tons of food we consume each year, the bulk comes from plants, which, with the help of sunlight, synthesize this food out of air, water, and soil. The remainder comes from animal products, which, in turn, are derived from plants. All the food, drink, intoxicants, and medicines that keep man alive ultimately come to us through the process of photosynthesis.[2]

Foods as Medicine

The idea that a plant contains powerful substances that can help heal infections, kill parasites, and thwart cancer is not new, just new to modern medicine. In traditional Asian medicine, foods and herbs have never been understood as separate and distinct; *both* are recognized for their healing properties. And two thousand years ago, Hippocrates said, "Let food be your medicine, and medicine be your food."

A vast new field of science is just beginning to scratch the surface of an understanding of the relationship between food and your health. Foods, these researchers are now finding, contain more than just vitamins and minerals. Almost every day there is a newly discovered "phytochemical" or "nutraceutical" found in fruits, vegetables, grains, herbs, and spices. These are substances naturally occurring in plants and foods that have physiologic activity but are not classified as drugs. What is coming to light is the nature of the vast chemical arsenal that plants have to help them survive the challenges of living and growing.

Our genetic makeup as humans has coevolved with our food supply. You have a direct, evolutionary, co-dependent, and intelligent relationship with your food. Plants have developed defenses and mechanisms in order to survive. This interdependency has been built into life on this planet since its beginning, as we can't make these "defenses" and "mechanisms" ourselves and thus are obliged to get them through our diet.

This chain of interdependency has been severely tampered with over the past fifty years. Every day, "commercial interests" are separating you from the natural interdependency built up over thousands of years. No synthetic food or drug can do the same complex job as its natural counterpart. A world of fast foods, plastics, pesticides, and additives has had a direct detrimental effect on the health of Westernized populations. Every day in the supermarket and in TV and radio commercials, one vested interest or another, with a product to sell you, places itself between you and the foods you need for optimal survival and health.

Consider the rise of the incidence of osteoporosis in our society. Before the refining of sugars and flours, osteoporosis was virtually unknown in Western culture, as were other degenerative diseases.[3] Osteoporosis is a disease of developed countries. The more you process food, the fewer minerals and nutrients you are getting in your diet, thereby breaking into that natural interdependency between nature's pure, unrefined food and your body. A diet high in protein, fat, and sugar will be low in all the trace elements. The pharaohs, when dug up, showed signs of osteoporosis, while peasant Egyptians did not. Ironically, the pharaohs' great wealth brought them a refined diet and a sedentary lifestyle, which leeched their bone mass and brought disease into their lives.

For Western women the incidence of osteoporosis is now extremely high. At age sixty, nearly 50 percent of American women will be diagnosed with osteoporosis—with the percentage increasing exponentially thereafter. In Asia, the incidence of osteoporosis among women is almost nonexistent. Women in those countries can live to a very old age without any sign of bone degeneration.

How can this be? We know that women in rural Asia are not taking calcium supplements. Nor are they popping Premarin. But there are significant dietary and lifestyle differences between Asian and Western women. Besides an absence of processed foods in their diets, Asian women eat much less protein, especially animal, and more vegetable and grains, affording them more minerals and nutrients. They eat plant foods high in phytohormones—such as tofu, miso, and other soy products. And the women in rural Asia don't have to concern themselves with bone loss because exercise is an integral part of their daily lives. Their traditional way of life has the benefit of giving them all the exercise they need to give their bones the stress necessary to keep them strong and healthy.

In chapter 11 we will discuss at greater length how a plant-based diet can have an impact on your health today and for the rest of your life, and how by eating a balanced plant-based diet, you can protect yourself from hormonal imbalances and osteoporosis. Our program will give you the best chance to keep breast and other cancers out of your life—without resorting to the drug therapy of companies motivated by finding new ways to sell you their products.

Plants and Healing

When a human body becomes "disordered" or "diseased," plants are the "healers" that humans have always relied on. Found in the grave of a Neanderthal man who lived over 60,000 years ago were seven species of medicinal plants—including ephedra, which is the basis of ephedrine, today a commonly prescribed drug.[4] If you've ever taken an over-the-counter asthma or cold remedy, you have used a synthesized version of ephedra. In fact, six of the seven herbs found in those Neanderthal graves are still in use today.

Healing Through the Ages

The healing methods of the ancient civilizations of Rome and Greece and medieval Europe consisted almost entirely of herbal medicine. *De Materia Medica (On Medicines)*, by the Greek herbalist Dioscorides, was Europe's first major herbal text and remained a standard reference for 1,500 years. After the invention of the printing press in the sixteenth century, *De Materia Medica* was one of the first books to be published. Though the Catholic Church came to officially view disease as punishment from God, to be cured by incantations and prayers, various orders of monks preserved the Greco-Roman herbalism by copying the ancient medical texts. In England, herbalism flourished. Culpepper's *Complete Herbal and English Physician* was first published in 1652 and has been in print ever since. The only medical work taken by the Pilgrim fathers on their voyage to the New World was a copy of Culpepper's book, and in the first 200 years of this country, the principle medicine practiced was herbal. In Colonial America, more women than men practiced medicine and relied on their time-tested herbal knowledge brought from the Old World, further enriched by contact with Indian healers. Male Caucasian practitioners of the period relied heavily on bleeding and the use of calomel (poisonous mercury).[5]

Herbs and Women: An Ancient Synergy

The link between women and herbs extends back to prehistoric times. In the early hunter and gatherer tribes, women were the gatherers and propagators of plants and traditionally cared for the sick, creating the earliest form of medicine: herbal. A Sumerian stone tablet from the third millennium B.C., considered the oldest medical document discovered, represents a figure known as Gula as the goddess of medicine during a period when most healers were thought to be women.

During the Middle Ages, male doctors trained mostly in theology in church-run universities wrested control of medicine from their herbally trained female counterparts. Women healers were pushed out by the guilds of physicians, surgeons, and apothecaries who served mainly the elite classes. Every country in Europe passed laws prohibiting the work of the women healers. Fueled by an infamous attack on women, *Malleus Maleficarum (Hammer of Witches)*, written by two German monks, and which became official doctrine in the Catholic church, from 1300 to 1650 a million or more women were burned as witches. The image of the folk herbalist was changed from wise woman to witch—another word for witch being "herbaria." The most damning accusation against a woman—besides "having intercourse with the devil"—was that she practiced herbal medicine. This nightmare period in Western history resulted not only in a senseless loss of life but was also a "holocaust" for plant medicine—the result was a great loss of valuable herbal wisdom.

This is not exaggeration. We know that centuries before Alexander Fleming "discovered" that a *Penicillium* mold killed bacteria, European peasant women bound moldy bread over wounds, and medieval wise women used ergot (a fungus that grows on rye) for labor pains and the plant belladonna to prevent miscarriage during a period when male practitioners were relying on bleedings and incantations. Ultimately, these herbal remedies were turned into drugs for profit, but the wisdom came from the folk medicine practiced for centuries. Fortunately, the witch hunts did not completely wipe out women's herbalism, which went underground. In England, for example, the "old woman" from Shropshire who helped popularize foxglove—source of the heart drug digitalis—said it came from a "secret family recipe."[6]

In the years following World War II, the "romance" of the U.S. medical community with synthetic drugs once again put plant-based remedies and tonics into disrepute. Before the war, drug companies were relatively small and unsophisticated "low tech" businesses that produced medicines to be bought largely over the counter. With the discovery of sulfanilamide, penicillin, and other antibacterial substances, there was an explosion of antibiotic products, and medicine entered a period of technological expansion in which the reliance on chemistry and machinery pushed aside the traditional use of herbal remedies. As noted in a 1967 *British Medical Journal* article, "Medical Science: Master or Servant?" by Lord Platt, "Modern medical treatment [often depends] on non-clinical, often non-medical scientists, frequently working in, or in close collaboration with the pharmaceutical industry."[7]

Whether you realize it or not, every pharmacy and hospital uses medicines derived from plant sources. Most of these medicines were revealed to pharmaceutical companies through the native wisdom of indigenous healers. Drugs like codeine, digitalis, quinine, and syrup of ipecac all contain plant products. In fact, drugs of plant origin still make up 25 percent of the drugs sold in the U.S. Drugs we take completely for granted, such as aspirin, were originally derived from a plant source. In Germany, where there is a greater acceptance of natural products for healing, drugs of plant origin make up 50 percent of the prescriptions written each year. (At the turn of the century, the number of drugs derived from plants was 50 percent in the United States as well, but the emphasis on manufacturing synthetics by the pharmaceutical companies has reduced this figure significantly.)

Herbs Specifically for Women

With present-day scientific analysis, we have learned that the traditional herbs used to ease feminine discomfort and to soothe the passage of menopause contain substances that are active in human hormonal systems. Some plants have components that correspond exactly to human hormones and others have substances that are not identical to our hormones but interact with and "auto-regulate" them. In fact, it's possible to say that "phytohormonal therapy" has been part of a "clinical trial" for women's discomforts for thousands of years.

These remedies can still work for you today. In the Natural Woman plan, we will discuss a number of traditional herbal remedies that you can use as a complementary or alternative program for midlife symptoms.

Among the ancient remedies with phytohormonal properties we will be recommending are:

***Cimicifuga racemosa* (black cohosh or squaw root):** A root used by North American Indians for balancing and normalizing female "hormonal" complaints. Today, the Enzymatic Therapy product Remifemin, which is based on *Cimicifuga,* is very effective for PMS and menopausal symptoms and is widely used in Europe. We will be recommending it as part of our plan.

***Angelica archangelica* or *sinensis* (dong quai):** Medical texts in China dating back 2,000 years describe *tang kuei,* as it is also known, as particularly helpful to women for problems relating to menstruation and for ensuring a healthy pregnancy and easy delivery. European *Angelica* was used over 1,000 years ago, and European colonists found *Angelica* being used by many Indian tribes.

***Dioscorea villosa* (wild yam):** The wild yam is mentioned for its healing power as far back as 25 B.C. in the *Pen Tsao Ching,* the most famous medical text in China, and was used for women's menstrual and menopausal difficulties. It was also used by Indian tribes in North and Central America.

***Vitex agnus castus* (chaste tree berry):** One of the most widely used herbs for women, it was well known by Grecian women and was a common remedy in medieval England. In ancient China it is mentioned in written texts going back thousands of years. North African women used it at least two thousand years ago.

And this is the short list. Many, many other plants, such as licorice, beth root, motherwort, red sage, sasparilla, fennel, and false unicorn root, have aided women through the centuries, and can still do so today. The knowledge of these plants and herbs has been handed down through oral and sometimes written tradition, in widely disparate cultures and vastly different time periods. In the nineteenth century, chemists used this "herbal convergence" to point them to plants that provided extracts for the first pharmaceutical drugs.[8]

The Modern Phytohormones for Women

As a result of modern chemical analysis and the discovery of new extraction techniques, a new plant resource for helping women balance and replenish their hormones has become available. Bio-identical estrogen/progesterone/testosterone hormonal products from the wild yam and soy can be synthesized in a laboratory. Plants contain substances that are precursors to human hormones and can be converted. These converted hormones go a step farther than the use of an herb known for its healing properties, or a food that when eaten has both healing and nourishing properties. Although these plant-derived hormones are synthesized in a laboratory and are not extracted from humans, they are *identical* to human hormones. They come in standardized dosages and are easily obtainable by prescription. In Europe, they have been available to women for over fifty years. *It is these bio-identical plant-derived hormones that form the basis of our hormonal replenishment plan.*

When asking for them, woman have started calling them "the naturals," and we are following that trend to easily identify them and to differentiate them from Premarin and other standard HRT products, which contain substances foreign to a woman's body.

You might ask what the difference is between a *synthetic* estrogen and estrogen that is *synthesized* from plants. It may seem confusing at first, but it is important to understand the distinction. A synthetic estrogen mimics estrogen but is not a substance that exactly matches human hormones and doesn't exist in nature. The plant-derived estrogen is created by a laboratory process but *exactly* duplicates your natural hormones. This exact matching means that "the naturals," when used in proper dosage, are free of harmful side effects, and are gentler and safer in every respect. Side effects from a drug occur when there is an imperfect match—like putting a square peg in a round hole. And it's not just that the synthetics don't fit, but they are also not metabolized as fast as bio-identical substances. Thus they linger in the body longer like an unwanted guest, sometimes landing on and stimulating hormone receptor sites other than the intended ones—all of which can increase your risk of side effects and cancer. We have been conditioned to believe that side effects are just an unfortunate but necessary part of taking "medicine," but this is rarely the case with natural plant-derived products. Premarin, which is created from horse urine and is sometimes referred to as *natural* because of this fact, contains horse estrogens, which do not match human hormones, along with other additives, which contribute to unwanted side effects.

In many ways, the use of "the naturals" represents a *modernized* return to the roots of an herbal tradition which, despite the mechanization of medicine and the reliance on synthetic drugs, has never entirely disappeared from use. We feel the pendulum is swinging back, as modern women can get the benefits of the foods and herbs that have been proven by time over thousands of years.

4

HRT: THE ROAD TO THE PRESENT DILEMMA

It's very difficult for a woman to make an informed choice if she must do so within the context of the false assumptions about hormones that have been built up over the last forty years. To be fully prepared to confidently make the right decisions for herself, a path needs to be cleared.

Because if it weren't for certain "accidents" of scientific discovery, and the roads chosen by pharmaceutical companies motivated primarily by profit, the majority of American women who need help in hormone balancing might today be happily availing themselves of the safe and effective natural estrogen/progesterone products, thereby bypassing altogether the darker aspects of HRT.

We believe that the HRT controversy is a false problem created mostly by persons with vested interests who have told women that when it comes to hormones, it's *either/or*: Do it their way or you can't do it. Live with the risks and side effects or you can't get any benefits.

Such black-and-white attitudes should always be viewed with skepticism because science is an ongoing process, not a fixed truth.

Think of how often yesterday's scientific wonder becomes today's discarded practice. Tonsils were routinely removed until medical researchers discovered their value and removal of them was discontinued. In the treatment of breast cancer, radical mastectomies were the standard until greater understanding proved that less extreme measures could be just as effective. Science doesn't proceed in a straight line, and the more it is driven by commercial interests that put profit to the forefront, the more likely it is to lead us seriously astray. In the case of hormones, scientific investigation has followed a zigzag course, dictated by a mix of accident, trends in scientific method, the profit motive, and quirky turns of fate.

Knowledge of Hormones Is Relatively New

The word "hormone" only came into the language as recently as 1905—from the Greek word meaning "urging on" or "roused to action"—so technical knowledge of how hormones work is still relatively new.[1] It was discovered that animal glands put out chemicals that are transported through the bloodstream like "messengers," and which then seem to tell the body's organs what to do. The early research on hormones was performed parallel with the beginning of an understanding of the female reproductive system, and in 1900, the role of the ovary was recognized in the hormonal control of the female reproductive system.

A form of estrogen was first isolated in 1923 by Willard Allen and Edward Doisy from the urine of pregnant women. They called it *theelin*; it was later called *estrone* (E1).[2] For obvious reasons, there was a difficulty in obtaining supplies.

Quite quickly, pharmaceutical companies, principally in Europe, realized that there could be a gold mine in this discovery of a female sex hormone, but the difficulty was in finding a method of production that would produce large quantities. In 1928, a German pharmaceutical company developed an injectable form of estrogen from human placentas, but the amount obtained from this source was still quite small. In 1929, the American scientists George W. Corner and Willard Allen discovered the corpus luteum, or "yellow body," which is formed in the ovary on the release of a mature egg. They were able at that time to extract a very small amount of progesterone from it.

In all these early studies, the animal research was severely inhibited by scarcity and prohibitive cost. Progesterone was so expensive to produce that even research scientists couldn't afford it. The minute amounts extracted from animals were quickly bought up to improve fertility in expensive racehorses. Only a few European pharmaceutical companies took the laborious steps of extracting hormones from humans and animals and converting them to usable form.[3]

Research emphasis on hormones was almost entirely on *animal* as opposed to *plant* studies, as the interest in plant medicine was essentially dormant during this period. The reasons for this are complex and beyond the scope of this book, but, briefly, after World War I, the expanding pharmaceutical industry moved away from plant extractions and toward "better living through chemistry." With a synthetic chemical compound, drug companies could obtain a patent on the end product and thereby have a chance of cornering the market. Research into plants could lead to the following dilemma: After spending considerable resources attempting to synthesize the active principle of a plant, the company might discover that it was too expensive a process for a product that could not be patented, or worse still, that it was less effective than the whole plant and thus worthless commercially.

In 1941, a pharmacologist writing in the magazine *Science* recounted that, "The desertion of the study of vegetable drugs soon became almost complete . . . Today is the heyday for organic synthetic chemicals. Present-day medical scientists only too frequently are apt to look askance at those who would investigate the therapeutic possibilities of the vegetable kingdom."[4]

In 1943, Willard Allen, working at the University of Washington in St. Louis, extracted an estrogenic product from horse urine. It proved plentiful and cheap to produce and had fewer side effects than previous extractions from animals. The patents for the "horse piss estrogen" or Premarin (for *pre*gnant *mar*e's ur*ine*) were sold to Ayerst Laboratories, ultimately providing the University of Washington at St. Louis with a very rich endowment.

This was a fateful moment for women everywhere. Like an invader without any resistance in the countryside, the Grand Army of Premarin would march into a vacuum. Backed by a formidable advertising arsenal, they overtook an essentially empty field. Other drug companies would enter the market, but Premarin would quickly gain a dominant position.

Feminine Forever: Selling the Concept of Sex Hormones

The early marketing of Premarin and other synthetic estrogenic compounds began when government monitoring of these products was negligible. Before World War II, drug companies were small-time concerns, making patent medicines that people could buy over the counter. The war changed all that. The development of sulfanilamide and other antibiotic products for the war effort created a rapidly expanding pharmaceutical industry that began to look everywhere for new markets.

Numerous new products that had undergone inadequate testing were introduced into the market—and tragedies ensued. Enovid and DES (*Diethylstilbestrol*), which was used extensively on pregnant women, were just two of the drugs introduced that turned into killers because of inadequate testing. And the thalidomide tragedy quickly forced the tightening of FDA controls, but the estrogenic drugs slipped through the cracks before these more stringent requirements were put in place. By the 1940s Premarin was regularly advertised in medical journals, with no restrictions on the claims made for it.

At first, Premarin was prescribed on a temporary basis for the relief of menopausal symptoms such as hot flashes, night sweats, depression, and vaginal dryness. But there were bigger mountains to climb.

Ayerst's most powerful salesman was Robert Wilson, M.D., a New York gynecologist. His 1966 book, *Feminine Forever*, written with the financial backing of the Ayerst laboratories, was the prime instrument for the promotion of the "horse urine" estrogen. As the leading proponent of menopause as an estrogen deficiency "disease," Wilson sought to save women from the loss of their "femininity" by putting them on a lifetime of Premarin. His promises sound quaint to today's ears and his "science" even quainter still. In *Feminine Forever*, for example, he counts the number of recipients of his estrogen replacement therapy as "between six and twelve thousand."

For a woman of the nineties, Wilson's book reads like an anachronism, as he was very much conditioned by the paternalistic culture he was reared in. Women were valued solely for their reproductive capabilities and their "femininity," by which Wilson meant their attractiveness to men. Once they stopped producing eggs, they seemed to lose all function in society.

"The unpalatable truth must be faced that all postmenopausal women are castrates . . . From a practical point of view, a man remains a man until the very end. The situation with a woman is very different. Her ovaries become inadequate relatively early in life. She is the only mammal who cannot reproduce after middle age," wrote Wilson. This is ludicrous. By this definition, women have only a *biological* purpose and no *social* purpose at all.

In fact, the wisdom and skills women accumulate beyond their childbearing years are, arguably, necessary from a biological and evolutionary point of view for the functioning of human societies. Medical anthropologists have pointed out that women have a stage at the end of their lives during which they cannot reproduce precisely so that they can rear their children to maturity before they die. Rather than being a negative or an aberrant trait, it is a uniquely *adaptive* one.

Though viewed as a crank by quite a few of his contemporary colleagues, Wilson, backed by the huge financial resources of drug companies, had the megaphone to himself. To give him the benefit of the doubt, he was perhaps carried away by a misplaced gallantry in his belief that he could rescue women and keep them "feminine forever." And let's face it, the positive estrogenic aspects of Premarin proved to be a big selling point. For the percentage of women who were able to take the drug without experiencing negative side effects, the estrogenic properties proved beneficial against the most common menopausal symptoms, not to mention the salutary effect of the belief that they could remain forever young.[5]

Feminine Forever sold 100,000 copies in seven months and was widely excerpted in women's magazines. By the early seventies more than 300 articles promoting the use of estrogen replacement therapy (ERT) appeared in women's magazines. By 1975, there were approximately six million women using Premarin in this country.

Then the boom was lowered. After a report of an increase in endometrial cancer among women at a Kaiser Permanente medical center in California, an article appeared in 1975 in *The New England Journal of Medicine.*[6] In it the researchers found that 57 percent of the women with cancer had used ERT drugs, whereas only 15 percent of the controls had done so. They concluded that the risk was increased by 7.6 times in women on ERT. And long-term users were at greater risk. Whatever the exact number of cases definitively linked to Premarin, women clearly died as a result of this early use of high-dosage Premarin.

Here we can see in stark outline the vast dangers of "medicine by advertising" as practiced in this country. When the primary driving force behind a drug is the expansion of the number of users, untempered by concerns for long-term effects and truth in advertising, the results can be devastating.

How ERT Became HRT

Enter Provera, otherwise known as *medroxyprogesterone acetate,* a completely new man-made substance never before encountered by the human body.

The early backfire in the use of Premarin did not send doctors away from the drug, and, in truth, it would have been a difficult task to induce women who had come to feel they needed Premarin to give it up. Instead, there was a period of retrenchment, and a new regimen was conceived. The dosages of Premarin were lowered, and based on studies showing that the addition of a synthetic progesterogenic substance, a *progestin,* decreased the likelihood of uterine cancer in women, those women with an intact uterus were given Provera with the Premarin. Women without a uterus, it was decided, didn't need the "protective" properties of progesterone, as lacking a uterus eliminated the risk of endometrial cancer. Which, of course, is true, but what about *other cancers?* And the necessary *balancing* effect of progesterone on estrogen? What about the other possible risks of unopposed estrogen? This arbitrary "edict" decided among a handful of physicians has become standard therapy.[7] In a later chapter we will talk about the need for progesterone among women who have had hysterectomies.

Meanwhile, there were significant problems with Provera.

For a large number of women, Provera is a bitter pill indeed. Gail Sheehy describes in *The Silent Passage* her nightmare ride on this drug. She writes: "The Provera was another matter. It brought on unbelievable physical and emotional symptoms I'd never experienced before. After a year of the combined hormones, my body seemed to be at war with itself for half of every month. My energy was flagging, and resistance to minor infections was falling. I felt as if I were racing my motor."

And that's not all. Beyond its numerous side effects, Provera interferes with your body's own progesterone production and may negate any assumed protective benefits of estrogen against heart disease.[8] Unlike bio-identical progesterone, the progestins such as Provera have been shown to attach to many kinds of hormone receptor sites—and the long-term effects of this action are just beginning to become known.[9] Provera's most negative side effect—the one that drives many women away from it almost immediately—is that it induces uterine bleeding. In other words, you continue to have a "period" for as long as you use it.

Despite what would seem daunting reasons not to risk it, Provera plus Premarin is still the regime most prescribed and recommended by U.S. medical doctors for a woman with an intact uterus.

In addition to the Provera "Band-Aid," the manufacturers of Premarin—reacting with entrepreneurial ingenuity to the drop in the sale of their drug following the "adverse publicity" of the cancer risk—launched a new campaign to reorient women to the need for their product.

Enter the idea of Premarin as a protector against osteoporosis. With the aid of a public relations firm, Burson-Marsteller, Ayerst Laboratories financed an extensive and expensive promotion in the form of articles in newspapers and magazines, print ads, and lecture tours of medical experts promoting the idea that "estrogen therapy" was the best protection against osteoporosis. Women who had never heard of *osteoporosis* were now being made aware of their dire need to protect themselves from it.[10]

The *actual* benefits of estrogen on osteoporosis were greatly exaggerated, if not misrepresented, and the existence of other protocols that are more effective and without the significant risks of Premarin (see chapter 5) were ignored, but this campaign proved extraordinarily successful, as evidenced by the fact that the use of Premarin for protection against osteoporosis is now deeply ingrained in the literature when the pros and cons of hormone replacement therapy are debated. But most of all, menopause has now become very big business. After a brief lull following the 1975 studies—when doctors pulled back from prescribing HRT drugs—sales of Premarin began to rise dramatically again, and it is now the number-one-selling drug in the country.

How Many Dead Horses for a Little Red Pill?

In 1995, Premarin sales reached 940 million dollars. Baby-boom women coming into menopause will add millions of potential customers. In light of these numbers, the methods of production of horse estrogen have come under serious scrutiny, and any conscientious woman should be aware of the manufacturing process before deciding to use the drug. Here, briefly, is how Premarin is produced:

A pregnant horse—we'll call her Patsy—stands on a concrete floor in a stall 8 feet long by 3½ feet wide. She is fitted with a rubber collection cup attached to a hose. For almost half of her eleven-month pregnancy, Patsy will stand on this concrete floor, unable to take more than a few steps in any direction as the narrowness of the stall prevents such simple movements as turning around and lying down. Allowing Patsy out to pasture might mean losing some of the urine dropping into her rubber cup.

After giving birth, Patsy gets a few months to pasture with her foal, during which time she is reimpregnated and then sent back to her concrete stall.

Her foals become the waste products of this process and are then "discarded." Some are killed immediately, others are kept as replacements for worn-out mares or to expand production; the majority are sold to feedlots to be fattened, then slaughtered for meat.

This procedure is what it takes to produce a Premarin pill. In 1993, *75,000* mares fitted with rubber collection cups stood on those concrete floors in those stalls. Since the beginning of production, we conservatively estimate that a total of 500,000 mares have performed in the service of Premarin, and over a million foals have been "discarded."[11]

If the Ayerst people keep up with the exploding baby-boom generation, to satisfy the market demand, *250,000* mares a year will stand in those concrete stalls located on *1,500* farms in the United States and Canada. This is deeply disturbing, especially in light of the existence of estrogen products from plants, which are more ethical, more economical, and more ecological, not to mention safer and more effective.

5

THE RISK/BENEFIT FACTOR

Once a woman has decided to consider replenishing hormones, either by her own choice or at the suggestion of her doctor, she will more likely than not be forced to grapple with the notion of the *risk/benefit factor* and the fear that can come with it. In order to make a completely informed decision on hormone replenishment, you need to understand why the risk/benefit factor as applied to Premarin/Provera need not apply to the use of "the naturals."

The Woman's Lonely Burden

While assessing one's risk/benefit factor may sound like good advice, in practice it is something else again. Most physicians put the onus of the decision to use HRT drugs primarily on the woman. Ultimately, she alone must make the choice by factoring in her present medical condition, her family history of disease, her reproductive history, her environmental history, and her psychological history. Quite a big job, and probably the least appetizing one she could imagine just when all the social and psychological pressure of discovering that she may be getting old come barreling in.

Let's try to break down the components of the risk/benefit factor for HRT. First, the possible benefits.

Benefits of HRT

Premarin (ERT) or Premarin/Provera (HRT) has been shown to mitigate menopausal symptoms such as hot flashes, night sweats, vaginal dryness, and depression, potentially to prevent Alzheimer's disease, and to provide antiaging effects such as smoother, plumper skin.

Heart disease is the leading cause of death for women in this country. Drug manufacturers and many doctors claim that taking HRT drugs protects a woman against the onset of heart disease. If they are correct, protection against heart disease is a benefit of HRT.

One in five American women will fracture a hip from osteoporosis in her lifetime, and 25 percent of these women will never walk again. Premarin has been shown in studies to slow the loss of bone in women with signs of osteoporosis if used over a period of time exceeding five years. Hence, prevention of osteoporosis is also presented as a benefit.

Risks of HRT

The risks of embarking on a long-term HRT regimen include the potential for breast cancer, endometrial cancer, ovarian cancer, blood clots, gallbladder disease, liver disease, and stroke. The most recent study as of this writing appeared in *The New England Journal of Medicine* in June 1995 and cited the increased risk for women on HRT for breast cancer.[1]

Also into the risk column go the side effects experienced by many women who take these drugs, such as weight gain, bloating, headaches, sore breasts, and depression, to give the short list.

Does HRT Protect Against Heart Disease?

Over and over, in countless books and articles about HRT, the benefits of HRT with respect to heart disease are taken completely for granted. If you go into Compuserve on your computer and check *Grolier's* encyclopedia under HRT, it states HRT's protection against heart disease as fact. At a recent large medical meeting, every physician in the room raised his or her hand in agreement when asked if HRT has been proven to prevent heart disease in post-menopausal women.[2]

Yet not all of the facts are in.

This is what appeared in an August 1995 UCLA Medical Center newsletter: After explaining that UCLA would be participating in the National Institutes of Health study of 160,000 women nationwide over a ten- to fifteen-year period, and that HRT's effect on heart disease in women was one of the issues to be studied, the principal UCLA investigator, Howard Judd, M.D., is quoted as saying, "If estrogen [he means here Premarin, which will be the drug used in the tests] does prevent heart disease, then that is an enormous benefit of hormone replacement, overshadowing every other reason to take it. Heart disease kills 250,000 American women a year, more than all forms of cancer combined."

In other words, according to this highly placed source, the jury is still out—way out—by ten to fifteen years on any definitively proven beneficial link between HRT and heart disease.

Despite this, on another page in the same newsletter in a column devoted to deciding whether or not to try HRT, women in menopause are advised to assess their long-term risks, and when deciding whether to pursue HRT are told to factor in the beneficial effects of HRT on heart disease.[3]

Confusing? Totally.

The 1995 Post-Menopausal Estrogen/Progestin Intervention study (PEPI) of 875 women in a clinical trial of three years reported that women on HRT regimes showed improved levels of the blood-clotting factor *fibrinogen,* in addition to raised HDL levels (the "good" cholesterol) and lowered LDL levels (the "bad" cholesterol). The authors of the study concluded that these changes are likely to be "clinically significant." The media then began to report this finding as proof that HRT prevents heart disease. Not so.

Lowering cholesterol is not the same as preventing heart disease. In fact, many other cholesterol-lowering drugs have been extensively studied and have not been found to reduce the risk of heart disease, and *some have actually increased the risk.*[4]

Even though ERT reduced the levels of the blood-clotting factor fibrinogen, that reduction did not appear to benefit anyone in the study. Ten women receiving ERT developed blood clots during the study, four of which were serious. In contrast, none of those in the placebo group suffered a clot.

Women who opt for ERT or HRT generally eat healthier food, exercise more often, and take better care of themselves, and, therefore, a reduction in heart disease risk may have nothing to do with hormone replacement.

So although prevention of heart disease is put in the benefit column, *a one-to-one correlation between taking Premarin and preventing heart disease is not only far from proven, it is highly questionable in the minds of a substantial number of critics of the studies.* Dr. Alan Gaby, who writes the column "Research Review" for the newsletter *Nutrition & Healing*, and one of the physicians highly critical of the conclusions of the PEPI study, points out that improvement in so-called risk factors such as cholesterol and fibrinogen levels does not necessarily translate into improvements in health, and he concludes that it is "quite possible that the medical profession is giving the wrong advice to women about estrogen therapy."[5]

Most important of all, what women aren't being told is that there are decidedly *better* ways to protect themselves against heart disease without putting other areas of their body at risk. Even women who've had complete hysterectomies and are considered more at risk don't have to resort to the HRT drugs for their only protection.

Even if we accept that Premarin/ERT does in fact provide protection against heart disease, if it is not the *only* way and there are equal or *better* ways to protect yourself, then this fact should be made part of any risk/benefit equation. Why include it as a benefit at all if there are better ways to protect against heart disease and the Premarin carries potential cancer risk?

For example, eating two cloves a day of garlic (or a garlic supplement) is also an excellent way to protect against heart disease without putting yourself in a danger zone. There are voluminous studies in the conventional scientific literature to show its beneficial effect in the prevention of heart disease.[6] Garlic not only reduces blood pressure, it also decreases cholesterol and the likelihood of internal blood clots—a triple threat to heart disease!

Plus, garlic has many other health benefits as well: There have been studies that suggest it can help prevent stomach cancer, strokes, and diabetes.

Garlic has what we would term "good/good" benefits. It gives you protection against heart disease, and it has no downside. ERT/HRT, on the other hand, has at best a "good/bad" benefit because of the substantial risk factor.

Your diet is a major factor in the prevention of heart disease. Dietary changes alone can provide the same effects on HDL and LDL cholesterol levels *without* the risks—and *with* added cancer protection. Many of the plants with phytohormonal properties have anticancer properties as well as benefits for your heart. Folic acid, the vitamin found in leafy green vegetables, significantly lowers the risk of heart disease.[7] The May 1996 *New England Journal of Medicine* details a large study on the protective values of vitamin E—found in vegetable oils and nuts, among many other foods—on your heart.[8] And soy, in particular, is powerfully beneficial to your heart.

Just losing weight will give you protection against heart disease. And exercise alone is one of the best protections against heart disease.

In other words, the best protection against heart disease for a woman without severe risk factors is a healthy lifestyle.

You are not a statistic. Advocates of HRT are fond of bringing forth the statistics about heart disease and osteoporosis when talking about why you should risk the HRT regime. This is how it's typically presented: Heart disease kills more women every year than all cancers combined. In 1992, 360,000 women died of heart disease as opposed to 43,000 from breast cancer. Ergo, the HRT promoters claim, all mature women need to protect themselves against heart disease with HRT drugs. Not only is there no proven benefit of HRT on heart disease, but even if there were, this constitutes an extraordinary leap in logic. What you are doing, in effect, is protecting yourself against a statistic! Turn this statistic around and you will see how absurd this thinking is. Consider the vast majority of women over fifty who *don't* die of heart disease. What did *they* do? To frame the reasons for taking HRT drugs in this way is to beg the question of why women are getting heart disease and osteoporosis in the first place. Why did all those

360,000 women die of heart disease? What were their individual risk factors? Their diets, their exercise habits, their genetic histories?

By taking HRT drugs all you may be doing is increasing by *one* the statistic showing how many women die of breast cancer—or uterine cancer, stroke, liver disease, and gallbladder disease, for which there is a statistical correlation with the use of HRT drugs.

HRT and Osteoporosis

Again, there exists a mass of confusion on this issue relative to taking Premarin or Premarin/Provera. In the most optimistic studies, the "estrogenic" properties of Premarin have been shown to *slow the loss of bone, but not to reverse the condition.* Even in the best of circumstances the effects on bone loss only continue for as long as you take the drug, and it must be taken long-term to have any positive effect. The dilemma here is that the longer you take the drug the more at risk you are for breast and endometrial cancer. In *Preventive Medicine Update* of September 1995, Dr. Jeffrey Bland states that American Home Products Company (makers of Premarin) are now considering backing off promoting Premarin for prevention of osteoporosis because of the concerns raised by studies of the drug that show that HRT must be used for the long term (at least seven years) to have *any* effect on osteoporosis at all.

There are now many doctors in the conventional and so-called alternative and holistic communities who tell women that the best ways to deal with heart disease and osteoporosis are through diet and exercise and natural hormonal balancing. In the chapter on preventing and reversing osteoporosis, we will tell you about the use of plant-derived natural progesterone to strengthen your bones.

In effect, the purported benefits of HRT drugs on osteoporosis and heart disease are so uncertain, so full of ifs, buts, and maybes, that to our minds HRT's role in preventing heart disease and osteoporosis cannot genuinely be listed as a benefit.

So what's left on the benefits side of the risk/benefit equation for HRT?

Purported Benefits of HRT	Risks and Side Effects of HRT
Mitigates symptoms such as hot flashes, night sweats Antiaging effects, such as smoother, plumper skin Mood elevation, greater alertness	Weight gain, bloating, headaches, sore breasts, depression, irritability, etc. With long-term use, potential for breast cancer, blood clots, ovarian cancer, endometrial cancer, gall bladder disease, liver disease, stroke

Does Premarin Alleviate the Symptoms of Menopause?

If the question is whether Premarin will control hot flashes and night sweats, the answer is yes, but at what price?

Will it mollify my mood? Will it soften my skin? Yes, but at what price?

The truth is that in all likelihood a very high percentage of the women taking Premarin do so for antiaging benefits, real or imagined. These are the same women who "won't give up their estrogen for anything."

If they are among that percentage of women who are able to tolerate the drugs without overly uncomfortable side effects, they get "hooked" on the positive benefits of the Premarin or Premarin/Provera regime and continue taking the drug because they feel it keeps them looking younger. They turn their minds away from the information about the risk of cancer and other types of disease.

It's certainly not surprising that so many women cling tightly to their "youth pills." Their doctors have urged them to do so for years, and as we've said earlier, the number of doctors recommending HRT for long-term use is increasing. The use of Premarin for its antiaging properties was promoted by many established physicians, one of whom, Robert Wilson, M.D., wrote the best-selling book *Feminine Forever*, which we mentioned earlier. But we think there are better, more acceptable sources for these benefits without the significant risk factors.

Still More Confusion from the Experts

In an interesting switch from decades of claims that Premarin was a miracle youth drug, members of the medical community now commonly insist that Premarin and other HRT drugs have *no effect whatsoever* on a woman looking more youthful. The *Berkeley Wellness Letter* of October 1995 from the University of California published the following, which begins by quoting an article in *Time* magazine:

> "America's No. 1 drug is an elixir of youth, but women must decide if it's worth the risk of cancer," *Time* told its readers. Actually, hormone therapy has never been an "elixir of youth," at least not outside the world of sensational best-sellers. It does not keep the skin young, act as a "tonic for the mind," make women feel "marvelous," or keep them lush, firm, and sexy, as *Time* claimed or implied.

With absolutely no data to back themselves up, the newsletter writers thus assert that HRT has no antiaging properties. But later in the same newsletter, the properties of estrogen and progesterone are described as important in their role "in building bone and other aspects of growth, in the condition of the skin and hair, and in behavior and brain function." The newsletter writers don't bother to explain why, when estrogen is taken as part of an HRT drug, it supposedly has no effect on these aspects of a woman's body. For twenty-odd years it was believed that HRT had antiaging effects. When was it decided, and by whom, that HRT had no antiaging effects? Were there studies done? We could find no such evidence anywhere. Most likely, this claim of no effect is a well-meaning but misplaced effort to discourage women from frivolously taking a drug with known cancer risks for its antiaging properties. The newsletter writers continue:

"Instead of mythology and wishful thinking, what women need is solid information. *But the facts are in dispute.*" [our emphasis] The newsletter then goes on to describe in detail the conflicting studies about breast cancer and HRT drugs . . . concluding with, "Where does this leave you? . . . Your decision about whether to begin, or continue, hormone therapy may now be more difficult than ever, and you will certainly need the advice of a physician . . ."

In sounding a clarion call for solid information, the newsletter writers follow a pattern we have seen everywhere in the menopause literature: There is great expounding on the existence of confusing data, and then even more confusion is added.

False Empowerment

In the guise of making women partners in important decisions about their health, doctors tell them they must assess their own risk/benefit factor. The trouble is, women are not being armed with solid information with which to make informed decisions. And decision making can get even more confusing when you factor in all the other possibilities when taking Premarin with Provera. Premarin plus Provera may increase the risk of breast cancer more than Premarin alone.[9] And there are studies which show that Provera can erase the benefit to the heart, which is not even a proven benefit to begin with![10]

In acknowledgment of the confusion surrounding the HRT drugs, women will also frequently be told that when taking these drugs they should be "closely monitored by a health-care professional." Though this may be well intentioned, it is to our mind a potentially dangerous palliative. Are these health-care professionals the same ones who are, to quote *Time* again, "giving out little red pills like M&Ms"? Or are they the ones who don't have time for the "emotional" complaints of their female patients? If these health-care professionals are subject to the same confusing information that women are, on what basis is it assumed that they will be able to *un*confuse it? Also, how does one "closely monitor" someone when it can't be known if you have a problem until you *really have a problem*: until you suddenly have breast cancer after fifteen years on HRT drugs. Sure, you can keep getting medical evaluations that will constantly put you in the doctor's office, but, ultimately, the onset of endometrial or breast cancer would remain fundamentally an *invisible* problem.

"Amid the current scientific uncertainty [about HRT], it's like betting all your money on a horse without knowing the odds for the race." This from an article in the conservative *Science News* in August 1995.[11]

A risk/benefit factor of the kind being proposed for HRT should apply only to those who are seriously ill. Then it makes sense. When applied to a basically *well* woman, it puts her in the position of deciding that in order to protect her heart and her bones, she must put her breast and uterus at risk. Put this way, it is starkly absurd. An essentially well woman with temporary menopausal symptoms is not the same as a woman with a life-threatening illness who is forced to put herself in the position of taking chances.

Modern medicine has a maddening tendency to treat women (and men as well) as part of a continuing drug experiment. The deaths of women from endometrial cancer due to the early use of ERT (Premarin) are chalked up to necessary casualties on the road of scientific progress.

What's a woman to do? Our advice: Get out of the "medicalized" game, which is so confusing that researchers can say in all seriousness that they hope to have some results for women by "early in the next century." Walter Willett, M.D., the lead researcher of the 1995 Harvard study that showed long-term use of HRT increasing breast cancer, is quoted as saying: "I am hopeful that by the time the current generation of young women approaches menopause, we will have alternatives for them."[12] So it seems that, until then, women are just on hold—until these doctors come up with something to save them.

Is a forty-five-year-old woman on the brink of menstrual change expected to put herself on hold while scientists conduct dueling tests? The PEPI trial and the Women's Health Initiative study are timed to give "answers" to women by the year 2005.

But What Answer Are We Waiting For?

These tests are using the same conjugated (mixed) estrogen compound (Premarin) and progestin that has already been shown to increase the risk of cancer with long-term use. "Conjugated estrogen [i.e., Premarin] and progestin are foreign to the human female: therefore, [these] reports should be regarded as a *toxicity* statement on a group of steroids possessing estrogenic, progestogenic, and/or androgenic activity." This statement is from Joel T. Hargrove, M.D., chief of Vanderbilt University's menopause center.

No More Ahead of the Game

Dr. Hargrove points out that the studies are specifically testing the Premarin/Provera regime and not "estrogen," or "progesterone." They are documenting the toxicity of these particular drugs, and, therefore, in 2005 we will just have more information about the Premarin/Provera regime *and be no more ahead of the game.* Dr. John Lee, the author of the recently published *What Your Doctor May* Not *Tell You About Menopause,* goes so far as to suggest that given the important distinction between bio-identical hormones and synthetic ones, all studies of the past that did not utilize bio-identical hormones should simply be discarded as irrelevant and useless.

We support Dr. Hargrove's suggestion that the most reasonable approach to testing should concentrate on the principal human female sex steroids (the ones that are made in a woman's body), estrogen and progesterone, providing measured levels of these native steroids. Dr. Hargrove then goes on to state that, in any case, "replacement with *natural hormones* which may be measured and maintained within a desired range of blood levels is a more rational approach for hormone replacement."[13]

We couldn't agree more. By following a program using diet, exercise, and supplements as the best way to protect against heart disease and osteoporosis, with the addition of "the naturals" for hormone replacement as needed, a woman can safely bypass the tyranny of the risk/benefit factor.

6

MORE THAN AN ALTERNATIVE

A woman could argue that Premarin/Provera, despite their risk factors and side effects, have been in use for forty years, and even if she does decide to use "the naturals," she might still have lingering doubts or questions. *Where do "the naturals" come from? How are they made? And, most important, just how safe are they?*

Most physicians and most of the lay public—assuming they are aware of their existence—harbor the misconception that *bio-identical plant-derived hormones* represent some kind of *new* treatment that has come from outside the mainstream, whereas the HRT drugs, principally Premarin and Provera, are the tried and true and the standard by which any other treatment should be measured.

But nothing could be further from the truth. In Europe (France and Germany, in particular), bio-identical plant-derived hormones from the wild yam and soy have been available since the late forties. In addition, they have been available in this country for nearly as long, but just not necessarily to you. In fact, when it comes to hormone treatment for women at midlife, to our minds what is now considered *conventional* should really be considered *alternative,* and what is *alternative* should really be considered *conventional.*

To understand why this is so, it is necessary to unravel the evolution of "the naturals."

The Scientist Who Synthesized "The Naturals"

As early as the 1930s, the American chemist Russell Marker became convinced that sex hormones could be produced from plants, some of which were known to contain steroid precursors, which could be chemically transformed into hormones. Many plants, principally *roots,* contain *sapogenin,* a variety of plant cholesterol that is structurally similar to human cholesterol, the building block of all hormones. Marker was a well-respected scientist, the man responsible for the discovery of a source of cortisone for the treatment of arthritis and whose concept of octane rating for gasoline is still in use today. He had noticed the work of German scientists in the field of plant steroids and had himself extracted progesterone from the urine of pregnant women—some thirty-five grams, which, at the time, was the largest amount ever produced in one lot. A Japanese chemist had given Marker a plant called *Dioscorea,* and Marker was struck by the ease of producing progesterone from its special variety of sapogenin, which its discoverers had named *diosgenin.*[1] Marker began looking at hundreds of possible plants for use in his experiments, the most promising of which was the Mexican yam (*Dioscorea mexicana*). His search for the *Dioscorea* that would prove to be the most abundant producer led him to Mexico and finally to the plant *Barbasco,* which, in his own words, was almost pure diosgenin.[2]

After lengthy studies, Marker concluded that he could convert diosgenin into progesterone by an efficient five-step process, which could easily be adapted for cheap mass production; a further three-step process would then convert it to testosterone; a further two-step process would convert it to estrogen.

The problem was that nobody believed him. The chemist Louis Feiser of Harvard University, the most respected authority in this field at that time, declared it impossible and said that nobody could do it. The head of Marker's department at Penn State had also declared it impossible. Marker wanted to do the work in Mexico, which is where the wild plants grew, and which he felt was the only practical location for reducing the huge mass of plant material into a substance that could fit in small bottles. Even after showing Parke-Davis, the pharmaceutical company funding his research, the large amount of progesterone he had extracted from his wild yam roots, he was turned down for additional funding. His superior at Parke-Davis declared categorically that no real scientific work could be conducted in Mexico. Whereupon Marker, a very stubborn and determined man, walked out of the company and the university and moved to Mexico City, where he set up his own laboratory in a tiny rented cottage. Following an adventure worthy of an epic film, he produced four and a half *pounds* of natural progesterone from his dioscorea—then worth eighty dollars a gram. This natural progesterone was worth over one and a half million dollars, an astonishing sum at the time.

From this remarkable beginning, Marker produced in a laboratory a *natural progesterone* that *exactly duplicated the progesterone produced in a woman's body.* With additional steps in the laboratory, it could be changed to *natural testosterone* and *natural estrogen.* But a direct road to producing a safe plant-derived hormone product for use by American menopausal women was not followed.

Why? For one, there was almost no interest in menopause in our culture at that time. On the whole, menopause was viewed as something that belonged in closed bedrooms with the blinds drawn. Women didn't talk about it among themselves. Many so-called "female complaints" around the time of midlife were either disbelieved altogether or were dismissed by the medical establishment as "emotional problems." It wasn't until Gail Sheehy's aptly titled book *The Silent Passage* was published that the intense glare of the media began to focus on menopause.

Enter "The Pill"

In the women's movement during the 1940s, the most pressing issue was birth control. Marker's breakthrough chemistry was immediately seen as vital to the production of a contraceptive pill, and the forces at work concentrated on that use for it.

Emphasis was placed on creating a synthetic progesterone product based on natural progesterone. The *half-life* of natural progesterone was very short—meaning that it left the body very quickly—so in order to create a substance powerful enough to break into a woman's cycle, researchers began experimenting with an agent that would give a longer half-life and would still produce or mimic the effects of progesterone. What evolved were very potent *progestins*—synthetic progesterones—which were powerful enough to prevent ovulation and accomplish the function of birth control. In fact, it was Marker's discovery that set in motion the production of what came to be known as "the Pill."[3]

Meanwhile, Marker himself had no sense of the wider possibilities for his discovery. He told an interviewer: "I was never interested in the use of the hormone, only in making it available. You just get curious and you want to see how the end comes out . . ." He said he didn't realize what it could be used for until years after his discovery. His terrible experiences with the commercialization of his product led him to quit chemistry for good in 1950.[4]

"The Naturals" Couldn't Be Patented

Marker did *not* apply for patents either in his own name or in a drug company's name, so the chemical process he devised was free and available to anyone to produce. He wanted to "leave the field open to anyone who wished to produce in competition, to force the price of the various hormones down to a point where they would be available for medical purposes at reasonable prices."[5] The great irony here is that this act of altruism on Marker's part had the effect of discouraging the U.S. drug companies from pursuing a natural source of bio-identical progesterone. It couldn't be patented; therefore, no one company could control the market.

This would prove to be a defining moment for women in this country. Unlike the situation with Premarin, where a patent could be applied for and the market controlled, no large pharmaceutical company in the United States picked up on natural progesterone preparations for use at midlife despite its many virtues and superior qualities (which are enumerated in the next chapter). One of the early deterrents to the production of natural progesterone was that at first it was believed that the only way to get enough into the body was to inject it, which could be painful. (The Eli Lilly Company has produced an injectable natural-source bio-identical progesterone for over forty years, but it has never been specifically approved or marketed for menopause.) Upon further study and attention, a *micronized* progesterone was formulated—meaning that the progesterone was reduced to very small particles—and it now can be taken quite easily in pill form. It can also be taken in a cream or gel (through the skin), or sublingually (under the tongue). But at the time, science and the country itself had embraced the "synthetics." Medicine was in the vanguard of the belief that the primary answers to the ills of society lay with technology.[6]

"Protecting" Women with Progestin

In 1977, when it became clear that unopposed estrogen in the form of Premarin could result in endometrial cancer, the decision was made to add a *progestin* to the ERT regime to protect the endometrial lining. At this point, progestins had been in use as a form of birth control for more than twenty-five years. To choose a progestin over natural progesterone for the purpose of protecting the endometrium was a highly arbitrary decision; most doctors believed at that time that the progestins worked exactly like natural *progesterone.* There was widespread ignorance about how a slight change in molecular structure could create a substance that could interfere with endogenous hormonal production. (Unfortunately, a survey of current medical literature shows that this error is still being perpetuated.) This estrogen/progestin combination is the conventional HRT in use today, mostly in the form of Premarin/Provera.

Unfortunately, the lack of clear information about the difference between progestin and progesterone has made many women prejudiced against *progesterone.* Even the typical physician still believes that progesterone and progestin have the same side effects. And Provera's serious side effects have prejudiced women against any form of hormone replacement.

"The Naturals" in the United States

Because of the dominance of the Premarin/Provera regime in the menopause marketplace, it is not well-known that the oral drug Estrace, and the patches Estraderm, Climera, and Vivelle, are based on *bio-identical plant-derived estradiol*. Estrace has been in use in the United States since 1976. The manufacturers of these estrogen products patented their delivery systems, which is one way to protect profit when using a natural substance as the primary ingredient. These plant-derived estradiol proprietary drugs are preferable to the Premarin/Provera regime. ("Proprietary" means exclusively owned and/or patented by a drug company.) They are not the drugs used in any testing of "estrogen," but were implicated by association in the cancer scare of 1977. Ironically, the *bio-identical* factor of Estrace, Estraderm, Vivelle, and Climera has never been promoted by these companies because, when they were first introduced, the romance in this country with synthetic drugs was in full swing, with synthetics holding sway over natural products and actually being considered preferable. Premarin is still the dominant estrogen product, and these other products represent approximately 10 percent of the estrogen marketplace, but now that our society has begun to understand the ill effects on health of pesticides, processed food, and other forms of synthetic adulteration, we may soon see changes in the way these manufacturers sell their products. In the Natural Woman plan, we will be recommending a combination of estrogens called tri-est (E1, E2, E3) over estradiol (E2) alone—the only form in which these plant-derived proprietary products are made.

"The Naturals" from Compounding Pharmacies

Since the early seventies, bio-identical plant-derived progesterone, estradiol, estrone, and testosterone have been available by prescription from compounding pharmacies. A compounding pharmacy goes beyond counting and packaging pills. It still does what all U.S. pharmacists used to do: actually formulate, or compound, drugs. Because of the domination of chain drugstores since the 1940s, the number of compounders steadily decreased in this country, and many people are unaware of their existence. With the new interest in unadulterated products—and not in small measure the interest in bio-identical plant-derived hormones—the number of compounding pharmacists is again increasing. There are now approximately 1,500 in the United States.[7]

If your doctor orders estradiol for you from a compounding

pharmacist, it would be the same basic product that is used in the estradiol proprietary drugs such as Estrace and Estraderm. We think the estradiol from the compounders is even more desirable because it doesn't have the additives—in the case of Estrace, binders and fillers; in the case of Estraderm, adhesive—but even these drugs would be preferable to horse-urine-derived estrogens or wholly synthetic estrogens.

A handful of large U.S. pharmaceutical companies manufacture the bulk of the bio-identical plant-derived hormones sold worldwide. Pharmacia-Upjohn, the largest in the United States, and Berlichem, a Schering-Plough subsidiary, are the major U.S. suppliers.

The fine chemicals division of Pharmacia-Upjohn has been processing plant-derived steroid hormones—progesterone, testosterone, and estradiol—which they make from soy—for over forty years. (Soy has a plant sterol similar to wild yams and is less expensive to produce.) Berlichem also produces estradiol, progesterone, and testosterone and is the only U.S. producer of estriol. (Diosynth in the Netherlands also supplies estriol to U.S. companies and compounding pharmacies.) Until recently estriol had a very small market here, but the Berlichem product manager supervising estriol sales recently told us that sales were increasing exponentially due to estriol's increasing use by women at risk for breast cancer or with breast cancer, for whom this estrogen is extremely beneficial.[8] This is a very good sign, and it shows the progress the use of estriol is making in this country.

And here is an example of a pharmaceutical company playing both sides of the market: Pharmacia Upjohn sells natural progesterone to the compounding pharmacies for their use, while at the same time selling natural progesterone to a sister division for its use in the *synthetic* progestin Provera.

Widespread Use of Bio-Identical Plant-Derived Hormones in Europe

In Europe, where pharmaceutical politics is played differently, quite a few companies began producing natural progesterone derived from plants back in the 1940s. The way medicine is practiced in Europe created a much more hospitable environment in which to follow up Russell Marker's breakthrough discovery. For one thing, plant medicine had never gone out of medical fashion in Europe, as it had in the United States. The major European pharmaceutical houses have traditionally sold both conventional pharmaceutical and herbal medicines side by side, and with an even hand. Fifty percent of their product production relies on herbal medicine.[9] Nor do the politics of patents drive the marketplace in the same way that they do in the United States. In a number of countries, drugs are price-subsidized by the government, giving less incentive to create drugs with "protected" profit.

Since the 1940s, bio-identical plant-derived *progesterone* has been in use in Europe for the treatment of PMS. Katharina Dalton, M.D., an English physician, pioneered this use of progesterone. Until Dr. Dalton's landmark work, PMS was not recognized as a real syndrome. Her dedicated fight, first to have PMS acknowledged, then to have hormonal imbalance seen as the primary culprit, and finally to show the benefit of progesterone in its treatment, was a long and difficult struggle. Now, of course, PMS is quite accepted by establishment medicine, but until the 1970s it was generally treated as a "mental" problem, if it was acknowledged at all. In her 1977 book, *The Premenstrual Syndrome and Progesterone Therapy,* Dr. Dalton spells out the safety record of natural progesterone: fifty years of continuous use in Europe and extremely safe.

What slowed down the wider use of bio-identical plant-derived progesterone for relief of menopausal symptoms was the belief that it could only be administered in suppository form. (Dr. Dalton herself believed this.) But this is no longer true, and the oral form of natural progesterone has been available for nearly twenty years.

Many European pharmaceutical companies manufacture both plant-derived estrogen and progesterone products. The French company Besins-Iscovesco makes Utrogestan, a progesterone capsule, and Oestrogel, an estradiol gel. Using a gel as the delivery system has been very popular in Europe and is only beginning to gain acceptance in this country. Oral micronized progesterone is available in France, England, and Germany. L. D. Collins Co., in Great Britain, makes Cyclogest, an estradiol suppository.

Estriol has been in use in Europe for half a century.[10] Many of the studies of its cancer-protective properties were done by European researchers, and because of its accepted safety there, it is used extensively as a vaginal cream. The large pharmaceutical company Organon, in the Netherlands, has been selling an over-the-counter estriol preparation called Oevestin for over twenty-five years.

Jumping on the Bandwagon

If you still harbor some skepticism about the plant-derived hormones, take this into consideration: Recognizing the growing demand for "the naturals," the major pharmaceutical companies are now jumping into this business in a big way. Novavax has received FDA approval to test its new product, Estrasorb, which would be the first U.S. proprietary drug to use a cream as a delivery system for natural estradiol. Schering-Plough is presently selling an oral micronized natural progesterone, Prometrium, in Canada. It has now applied for FDA approval to sell it in the United States. Johnson & Johnson has been researching the possibility of introducing an over-the-counter progesterone product. Wyeth-Ayerst and Columbia Industries have formed a partnership to distribute the drug Crinone, which is a vaginally delivered natural progesterone. Their joint press release declares: "Natural progesterone is superior to synthetic progestins which have been associated with side effects. Additionally, direct delivery to the uterus allows the therapeutic effects to be maximized while avoiding high systemic concentrations and side effects."[11]

However, this same company, Wyeth-Ayerst, just introduced Prempro—Premarin plus a *progestin*—which, in the press release mentioned above, is associated with negative side effects. Here is but another example of the large drug companies playing all sides of the market to their own advantage and adjusting their strategy when a demand arises.

Ultimately, it is women and their doctors who must decide on the best treatment. If doctors allow the drug companies to dictate treatment, they are doing a disservice to their patients. If women don't think for themselves—and, if necessary, educate their doctors—they can be subject to spectacular mistreatment. Think of those early women who used Premarin at high doses and ended up with endometrial cancer. The large pharmaceutical companies produce beneficial products, but we have all witnessed what can happen if decisions about treatment are left primarily in their hands.

Fortunately, even the most entrenched treatment protocols can change dramatically in just a few years. We are heartened by a recent medical story about Barry Marshall, M.D., a lone Australian practitioner who single-handedly turned around the ulcer business. The belief that ulcers were caused by excess stomach acid was dogma in the conventional medical profession, with reams of technical papers, textbooks, and, of course, a *billion-dollar industry of acid-blocker drugs* behind it. It was a proven, accepted fact. Barry Marshall showed definitively that most ulcers were not caused by excess stomach acid and were primarily activated by a bacteria. All the previous literature was upended, and what was once absolutely "medically true" was no longer so.

Here in the United States, the upending of the standard HRT regime is being driven by women. They are demanding better treatment, demanding answers. Within two years, we predict that you will have your choice of a custom-tailored estrogen/progesterone product from the compounding pharmacies, or newly marketed ones from the proprietary drug houses, once these products have been approved.

Listen to the testimony of compounding pharmacists:

> "Everyone wants 'natural' as opposed to synthetic. Growth is exponential and word of mouth is definitely the biggest factor."

> "Women are not just telling one or two other women, they are telling ten to twelve other women, and they in turn are telling twenty other women. . . . Doctors are being forced to pay attention because women are bringing them the solution [to negative side effects]. They are demanding better treatment. Some doctors are happy, but many of them are angry. . . . "

> "In terms of safety and efficacy, there is no comparison [of the naturals] with the synthetics. The biggest problem we experience is that women who were taking Premarin/Provera can't

understand why their insurance companies are not yet accepting the 'naturals,' and they are upset about it. We get dozens of phone calls a day—three fourths are from doctors wondering what's going on. Their patients are demanding answers and they [the doctors] are being forced to deal with it. Most of the doctors get their information from pharmaceutical reps. They [the doctors] say they want to see the research but they never read what we send them. The age of the doctor is relevant: Younger ones are more open; the older ones are more stuck in their ways."[12]

7

"THE NATURALS": WHAT ARE MY CHOICES?

Once a woman has committed to use "the naturals" for hormone replenishment, she might ask, *How do I choose among them? What's available, and what do I ask for when I talk to my doctor?*

In Part Two, we will give you specific recommendations for your personal midlife profile, but here we are presenting an overview of the bio-identical plant-derived hormone combinations that are available to women in this country.

There are two basic ways in which to get plant-derived hormones for yourself: in preformulated packaged products or from compounding pharmacies. The majority of women using "the naturals" obtain them through their doctors by prescription from compounding pharmacists who make them to order. Only estradiol (E2) is now in proprietary drug form. (In appendix B we will supply you with all you need to know about the compounders.)

Since we believe that progesterone is just as important as estrogen in hormone replenishing treatment, we don't recommend taking estrogen alone for symptom control—even if it is plant-based and even if a woman has had a hysterectomy. Besides balancing the effects of unopposed estrogen, such as water retention, progesterone has other vital functions. Like almost all hormones, these two work on an *axis* system—that is, they are *designed* to work in tandem.

There are four basic prescriptions for "the naturals":

Progesterone alone.

Tri-estrogen (E1, E2, E3) plus progesterone. E1, E2, and E3 in this formulation are in a one-one-eight combination—that is, one part estrone and one part estradiol to eight parts estriol—a formulation that was modeled offering the ratio of the stronger estrogen-stimulating effect of estrone (E1), estradiol (E2) in lower amounts with the protective, weaker estriol (E3) in higher amounts. (The estrogenic potency of estradiol is twelve times that of estrone and eighty times that of estriol.)[1] Recently, some physicians have begun prescribing bi-estrogen, which is 80% estriol and 20% estradiol.

Estradiol (E2) plus progesterone. A number of M.D.'s and complementary medicine practitioners use estradiol (E2) plus progesterone instead of the tri-estrogen formulation.

Estriol (E3) plus progesterone.

The means by which a substance enters your body is called a *delivery system.* In the case of "the naturals," there are a variety of ways in which the hormones can be formulated: pill form, drops, sublinguals (dissolved under the tongue), cream, gel, vaginal or rectal suppositories, and injection. In the Natural Woman plan, we will be recommending *creams* and *gels* as the first line of delivery, followed by delivery in pill form.

Are "The Naturals" FDA Approved?

It is a common misunderstanding among conventional doctors that somehow "the naturals" do not have the same FDA approval as do the proprietary conventional HRT drugs, but they do. Only in the case of *estriol* is there some disparity in the *level* of FDA approval.

The proprietary drugs Estrace, the patches Estraderm, Vivelle, and Climera—which are based on the plant-derived estrogen estradiol, with the addition of a patented delivery system—have specific approval for menopausal indications. Since the primary ingredient and source of the estradiol as compounded by pharmacists is identical to Estrace and the patches, this extends approval, per FDA guidelines, to the compounded plant-derived estradiol for menopausal symptoms.

Natural progesterone and Provera (and other progestins) have the exact same level of FDA approval—that is, *neither* is specifically indicated for menopause, but can be prescribed by your doctor for its indications. To put it another way, the bio-identical plant-derived progesterone, either sold by Eli Lilly & Company for injectable use, or compounded into gels, pills, creams, or sublinguals by the compounding pharmacies, and Provera, the progestin synthesized from bio-identical plant-derived progesterone, *have the exact same status vis-à-vis the FDA*: That is, they are specifically indicated for: "secondary amenorrhea (absence of menstruation); abnormal uterine bleeding due to hormonal imbalance in the absence of organic pathology, such as fibroid or uterine cancer."[2] Doctors can then prescribe these products for menopausal indications. This is a common practice called "offlabel usage"—that is, prescribing a drug for something it has not been approved for but for which it has been found to be beneficial.

Plant-derived estriol, which is identical to human estriol, has met the strict standards for products sold in the country set by the U.S. Pharmacopeia, the organization that sets the official standards for medical products used in the U.S. Estriol is not specifically approved for particular medical indications, but it can be legally prescribed for you by your doctor. No U.S. drug company that we know of has ever applied for FDA approval of an estriol product, but given the marked increase in orders reported by Berlichem, the division of Schering-Plough that sells the products, change may be on the way in this regard, which could accelerate widespread acceptance and help women in need.

Let's consider the benefits and drawbacks, if any, of the four most commonly prescribed combinations of "the naturals":

Progesterone (Alone or in Combination)

Progesterone is known as a *precursor* hormone for other hormones, which means that the body uses progesterone to create *other* hormones, such as estrogen, testosterone, and the adrenal corticosteroids. Seen in another way, the body can direct and control the production of other hormones by using progesterone as its source. The body can often balance any deficiencies or excesses of other steroid hormones in this manner.

This is an extremely important function, one that progestins cannot duplicate. Progestins *occupy* (take over, so no other substance can use them) progesterone receptor sites, interfering with progesterone *precursor* functions; they are also difficult for the body to metabolize and excrete. They cannot help our bodies balance or produce other hormones as needed.

Among its numerous benefits, bio-identical plant-derived progesterone:

Doesn't interfere with the body's own production of progesterone, as do the progestins. The progestins actually lower your body's own progesterone levels.

Exactly duplicates your body's own progesterone.

Helps balance estrogen, which a progestin cannot do.

Leaves the body quickly, like your own native hormones. The progestins remain in the body longer—thereby occupying receptor sites.

Can be more *consistently utilized* by the body.

Can *improve sleep.*

Has a *natural calming* effect during the day.

Helps *balance fluids* in the cells. (When used for PMS, bio-identical plant-derived progesterone can eliminate water retention and weight gain. It does the same when used for peri-menopausal or menopausal symptoms—that is, it balances out the properties of estrogen.)

Appears to have a *positive effect against hypertension.*[3]

Improves the body's ability to use and eliminate fats. This is a very important benefit for the midlife woman, because the body's ability to perform this function lessens with age.

Is superior to Provera in its effect on cholesterol per the PEPI study.[4]

Promotes new bone formation. A number of recent studies indicate that, unlike estrogen, which has so far only been shown to *retard* bone loss, progesterone can *stimulate new bone* and can be an important treatment for osteoporosis.[5]

May protect against breast cancer. The most important human study, reported in the *Journal of Fertility and Sterility,* April 1995, shows definitive evidence of bio-identical plant-derived progesterone's ability to inhibit estrogenic stimulation of normal breast epithelial cells. In other words, it has proven antiestrogenic effects, therefore demonstrating potential cancer protection. There is also evidence that when applied directly to the breasts, bio-identical plant-derived progesterone offers protection against estrogen-stimulated cell proliferation (called hyperplasia)—which can lead to cancer.[6]

Normalizes libido. There is evidence that it is progesterone (along with testosterone) that is most responsible for a healthy sex drive. The fact that many pregnant women report heightened sexual desire can be attributed to the increase in progesterone secretion during pregnancy. A 1994 animal study demonstrated that progesterone stimulated sexual activity.[7]

Regrows scalp hair. Women who have experienced hair thinning as a midlife symptom can reverse this trend by using natural progesterone.

Bio-identical plant-derived progesterone has none of the side effects of the progestins. A small number of women on initial use have paradoxical reactions, such as agitation and breast sensitivity, but these symptoms go away quickly. This temporary phenomenon is caused when estrogen receptors become temporarily sensitized to the addition of the progesterone. When the body adjusts, the symptoms disappear. Drowsiness can also sometimes occur, but can quickly be eliminated with dose adjustment.[8]

The Progestins: Risky Business

As we've already said, progestins came into being with the invention of the birth control pill—altered and hyped up so as to interfere with ovulation. They are many times more potent than natural progesterone. Among the most serious of their negative side effects:

- Lower your body's innate production of progesterone.
- Exacerbate a hormone imbalance leading to mood swings, headaches, fluid retention, and weight gain.
- Some of the progestins also have masculinizing effects, such as growth of facial hair and acne.
- Can cause blood clots.
- If used during pregnancy, can cause birth defects.

The 1995 PEPI study showed that Provera protects the endometrium from the build-up of cancer cells, but at what cost? Bio-identical plant-derived progesterone does it as well, and without Provera's undesirable side effects.

The Tri-Est (E1, E2, E3) Formula

Tri-est, as it's called, is one part estradiol to one part estrone to eight parts estriol. It was developed by Jonathan Wright, M.D., who has been prescribing estriol since the 1980s. By adding the smaller amounts of the "stronger" estrogens—estradiol and estrone—to the formula, symptoms such as hot flashes and night sweats could be alleviated more quickly, while at the same time giving a woman the potential protection against breast cancer of the estriol. The tri-est formula has been gaining in popularity over the last five years. Some pharmacists believe that with more fine tuning, and monitoring of blood levels, this formula can be adjusted even further to a woman's particular needs, for example, 1.25 to 2 to 8.

We believe that using a tri-est formula is good commonsense for women who want or need to use an estrogen product. Unlike Premarin or synthetic estrogens, it contains the three major estrogens (E1, E2, E3) in a balanced ratio that is more similar to a woman's own ratios. There is a body of scientific evidence that supports estriol (E3) as being non-carcinogenic, and even anti-carcinogenic. All the answers aren't in yet, but it's clear that with proper dosing, estriol has by far the least carcinogenic potential of the estrogen products currently marketed. Using tri-est, you are able to influence a greater number of estrogen receptors with safer, more benign estrogen. While there is a great deal of documentation on the tissue-stimulating effects of Premarin and estradiol alone, we know of no documentation that shows that estriol taken appropriately stimulates endometrial (uterine) cell growth, a precancerous condition. Overall, the tri-est formula gives you the benefits of estrogen without unnecessary health risks.

The only drawback to using tri-est is that it may not be a strong enough formula for some women at certain times, such as immediately following a hysterectomy.

Plant-Derived Estradiol (Plus Progesterone)

Although we recommend using the tri-est formula plus progesterone, or estriol plus progesterone, as a first line of treatment for most women who fit the model for estrogen replacement, the combination of bio-identical plant-derived estradiol (E2) plus progesterone is preferred by some doctors who advocate and prescribe "the naturals." Joel Hargrove, M.D., head of the Vanderbilt University Menopause Center and a leading M.D. advocate of "the naturals," published a study in the *Journal of Obstetrics and Gynecology* in 1989 that followed a group of women using oral micronized estradiol and progesterone. The study showed the superiority of this treatment over Premarin/Provera—it had all the benefits of Premarin and none of the negatives. And it included an added benefit: Two patients in the study who had evidence of fibrocystic changes in their breasts at the onset of the treatment showed definite improvement at the completion of the study. Dr. Hargrove has recently done an expanded follow-up study, which further confirms the findings.[9]

Because of the cancer-preventive benefits of the estriol, we believe using the tri-est formula should be a woman's first choice over estradiol, but some women may need to work with estradiol/progesterone to get sufficient symptom control. And in the case of women who've had a hysterectomy, it may very well be necessary to begin with a course of estradiol plus progesterone to get the initial effects of the stronger estrogen, at least in the short term.

Estrace, and the patches Estraderm, Climera, and Vivelle, are the proprietary drugs based on estradiol; your doctor can also prescribe a custom dose from a compounding pharmacy.

Estriol (E3) (Plus Progesterone)

Estriol (E3) is the estrogen that is made in large quantities during pregnancy. It is made by the placenta when the ovaries are "resting."

Both estriol and progesterone, which predominate over the other sex hormones in pregnancy, have potential *protective* properties against the production of cancerous cells. Women who have had numerous abortions without carrying a pregnancy to term are known to have an increased risk of breast cancer. This fact is proved very intriguing to many researchers, who speculate that the reason for this is that these women experience *reduced exposure to the protective estrogen, estriol.*

Estrogens, in general, tend to promote cell division, particularly in hormone-sensitive tissue such as the breast and the uterine lining. Of the three estrogens, estradiol is the most stimulating to the breast, and estriol the least. Estradiol is 1,000 times more potent in its effects on breast tissue than estriol. Studies of two decades ago clearly found that *overexposure to estradiol* (and estrone, to a lesser extent) *increases one's risk of breast cancer, whereas estriol is protective.*

An important 1966 *Journal of the American Medical Association* article by H. M. Lemon, M.D., reported a study showing that higher levels of estriol in the body correlate with remission of breast cancer. This finding is a potential boon for women at risk for breast cancer. Dr. Lemon demonstrated that women with breast cancer had reduced urinary excretion of estriol. He also observed that *women without breast cancer have naturally higher estriol levels,* compared with estrone and estradiol levels, than women with breast cancer. Vegetarian and Asian women have high levels of estriol, and these women are at much lower risk of breast cancer than are other women. Estriol's anticancer effect is probably related to its antiestrone properties—it blocks the stimulatory effect of estrone by occupying the estrogen receptor sites on the breast cells.[10]

In fact, *estriol has been used as a treatment for breast cancer.* A. H. Follingstad, M.D., presented results in *The New England Journal of Medicine* of a study in which small doses of estriol were given to a group of post-menopausal women with spreading breast cancer, and 37 percent of them experienced a remission or arrest of their metastatic lesions. There have been recent reports that it is better than tamoxifen for women with breast cancer.[11]

Estriol is the estrogen most beneficial to the vagina, cervix, and vulva. In cases of vaginal dryness and atrophy—which predisposes a woman to vaginitis and cystitis—topical estriol is the most effective and safest estrogen to use.

Estriol is better than estradiol for the treatment of urinary tract infections.[12]

Estriol has the benefits of the stronger estrogens without the risks. A study followed twenty women, ages forty-four to sixty-two, for two years on two milligrams of oral estriol. Within three months 86 percent of them showed improvement in menopausal symptoms, as well as reductions in vaginal atrophy. Another study followed the cardiovascular condition of post-menopausal women using estriol and found increased cardiac function, with improved blood flow in the extremities. [13]

Estriol leaves the body more quickly than estradiol and estrone, which is why it is sometimes referred to as a "weak" estrogen. In effect, it "grazes on" the receptor sites, delivers its message clearly and accurately, then quickly moves off. You do have to take a higher dose: For a dose equivalent to 0.6 to 1.25 milligrams of Premarin you would require 2 to 5 milligrams of estriol. But this so-called weakness is a benefit, because the higher a woman's estriol level, the less likely she is to get breast cancer!

Estriol treatment results in the reemergence of friendly lactobacilli bacteria and the near elimination of pathogenic (undesirable) colon bacteria, as well as restoration of normal vaginal mucosa and resumption of normal low ph.[14]

Estriol can prevent bone loss in postmenopausal women (see p. 168).

If Estriol's Benefits Are So Great, Why Isn't It Used More?

We predict that many years from now medical historians will be shaking their heads over the difficulty that estriol had in gaining full acceptance in this country. But *estriol cannot be patented.* Given the influence of the pharmaceutical industry over medical practitioners and the industry's vested interest in maintaining the preeminence of the HRT drugs already in the marketplace, there is a considerable drag effect, to say the least, in getting estriol to the attention of doctors. This, despite its proven track record in Europe as both a prescription drug and an over-the-counter product. Its safety record is excellent.

And there are, in fact, many U.S. doctors crying out for estriol's acceptance in this country. The most well-known article on the subject, by A. H. Follingstad, "Estriol, the Forgotten Estrogen," in *The Journal of the American Medical Association* (1978), made an impassioned plea for estriol's use. Dr. Follingstad blamed the FDA for blocking the use of estriol by requiring extremely expensive tests of efficacy. "Do we as clinicians have to wait the years necessary for the completion of these trials before estriol becomes available to us? I think not. Enough presumptive and scientific evidence has been accumulated that we may say that orally administered estriol is safer than estrone or estradiol."[15]

The key question is this: Given the strong evidence that unopposed estradiol and estrone may cause breast cancer, and that estriol and progesterone, the two major hormones produced throughout pregnancy, *are protective against breast cancer,* why aren't these two beneficial and safe hormones used routinely for women whenever hormone stimulation is indicated?

Estriol Is Gaining Ground

Our survey of the major compounding pharmacies showed that the use of estriol is rapidly gaining ground. The biggest hurdle to even greater acceptance is education: separating estriol out from the pack, so to speak, in order to help women and their doctors understand its *unique* properties, especially the fact that it can be a great boon to women at risk for breast cancer or who have suffered from breast cancer.

The ultimate goal is to get women to use hormone replenishment products with the greatest efficacy, in their most beneficial quantity, in their *purest* form in terms of chemical makeup, and in their *purest* delivery system.

8

TALKING TO YOUR DOCTOR ABOUT "THE NATURALS"

It may not be easy to find a doctor who already prescribes "the naturals" or one who is willing to learn about them, especially for women who live outside major urban areas. There would be less need for this book if that were so. Even though "the naturals" in a variety of forms are available through licensed pharmacists and can easily be prescribed for you by your doctor, he or she may still resist doing so. In Part Two, we will guide you to the resources available to help you locate a doctor who uses "the naturals," but in order to be a strong advocate for yourself you need to understand why you may encounter surprising resistance.

Beyond the fact that your doctor may have no knowledge of these remedies, his or her fear of malpractice suits can work against your getting proper treatment. It is a fact of our medical system that it is safer for an M.D. to prescribe a drug considered to be "standard"—even though the doctor may personally question its usage—than to prescribe a medicine that has been shown to work for decades but is not a part of "standard medical practice."

John Lee, M.D., a leading researcher on the use of bio-identical plant-derived progesterone, wrote in *The Multiple Roles of a Remarkable Hormone* in 1989:

> Few people know that the definition of malpractice hinges on whether or not the practice is common among one's medical peers and has little (usually nothing) to do with whether the practice is beneficial or not. A doctor willing to study, to learn the ins and outs of an alternative medical therapy, and to put what he has learned into practice in helping patients is potentially exposing himself to serious charges of malpractice . . .
>
> U.S. physicians are the captive audience for pharmaceutical advertising. They learn which drugs to prescribe. They do not learn of alternative and perhaps better ways of treating illness. If one were to seek this information for himself, he finds himself out of the realm and benevolence of his professional guild. Further, he is reluctant to be perceived as practicing in a manner different than his peers not only because of his fraternal associations with men but also because of the threat of malpractice charge, however unfounded.
>
> Thus, when he hears of the uses of *natural progesterone*, he wonders why none of his associates know about it. . . . I have observed numerous instances wherein perfectly fine physicians will inquire about obtaining the product [natural progesterone] for use by their wives or mother-in-law but not for their patients. What can account for such behavior by professionals? . . . I suspect it is fear of alienation from the flock that is paramount in their minds.[1]

That, and those daunting words: not an FDA-approved drug.

FDA Approval

Although "the naturals" are FDA-approved substances and can be prescribed by your doctor for the same indications as the proprietary drugs if they contain ingredients equivalent to approved drugs, they are not approved *proprietary drugs.*

In order to understand the distinctions, it is necessary to ask the question: What, exactly, does FDA approval mean? Are drugs that pass muster with the federal Food and Drug Administration guaranteed to be safe, and are drugs that lack approval automatically harmful?

A common misconception is that the FDA uses its own laboratories to test drugs for safety. What actually happens is that drug companies test their own drugs, then submit the results to the FDA. Then, through a series of steps, the FDA reviews the drug company's data and passes judgment. Unfortunately, this is a method with an enormous potential for abuse. There is abundant evidence of drug companies misrepresenting results and withholding evidence of side effects.[2] After all, the stakes are extremely high. The average cost of testing a single drug is now *250 million dollars.*[3] The potential rewards of gaining approval for a drug run into the billions of dollars.

So if you've got a hundred million or so to test a remedy, you can get the highly prized FDA approval for your drug.

But that doesn't mean that what is out in the drug marketplace as *FDA approved* is necessarily the most effective or safest treatment. It is, fundamentally, a treatment that the drug company wants to sell you!

In an ideal world, an FDA-like agency would carry on tests that would help women (and men) discover the safest, most effective, and most economical remedy available for a problem. But this is not how it works in practice.

If you are selling a natural remedy used successfully for two thousand years by Asian women—a pretty substantial human study in our opinion—this remedy would not at the present time be approved by the FDA for a specific medical use. Take the cases of ginseng or dong quai: The safety and effectiveness of these remedies may be supported by individual studies and clinical usage, and they have been shown to be effective, but they will still never get the stamp of FDA approval—unless someone can come up with the millions of dollars that it would take to pass through all the approval hurdles.

Therefore, the remedy can carry the curse of *not FDA approved.* Which doesn't mean it can't effectively treat your problem, doesn't mean it hasn't worked for hundreds, even thousands, of years, doesn't mean it can't be prescribed by your physician; it may just mean that this remedy hasn't passed through the FDA's bureaucratic system.

In his book *The Good News about Women's Hormones* (Warner Books, 1995), Geoffrey Redmond, M.D., an endocrinologist who otherwise seems to share the conventional physician's angst about natural products, says the following:

> Why not use progesterone itself (instead of Provera, a synthetic version) . . . Wouldn't this be more logical? . . . Some believe that it is. Micronized progesterone preparations need to be ordered from a pharmacy that makes them. Because progesterone itself is not patentable, the major pharmaceutical companies have so far not been willing to spend the money necessary to develop a natural progesterone preparation. This means that progesterone is available only to women who are able to make the effort to find a pharmacist who can supply it . . . *This is truly unfortunate* [our emphasis] because many women do feel better on progesterone than on MPA (Provera, Cycrin), etc.[4]

Gail Sheehy reported on this phenomenon from the front lines in *New Passages*, published in 1995:

> In the first edition of *The Silent Passage,* I reported that new-generation gynecologists and research scientists, such as Dr. Jamie Grifo at New York Hospital–Cornell Medical Center, believed the wave of the future to be natural micronized progesterone. It is widely used by European women. But American physicians have been reluctant to prescribe it because it doesn't have FDA approval [as a drug]. Our medical-pharmaceutical establishment persists in fostering suspicion of any "natural" compound that might alleviate symptoms, a shaky position given the many "natural" plants and tree barks from which major drugs like digitalis and even aspirin are derived.
>
> The investigators for the Postmenopausal Estrogen and Progestin Interventions study (PEPI), the three-year government sponsored study, did not share this outmoded view . . . Their boldness paid off in the good news when the results of the three-year study were announced in late 1994. Estrogen [in this case Premarin] combined with *natural progesterone* turns out to be the

> best regimen for a woman with a uterus. . . . There was only one problem. American women can't get natural micronized progesterone.
>
> Schering-Plough, the German company that supplied it to the PEPI trial for experimentation, *sells the product in Europe* [our emphasis] but did not apply for FDA approval and thus cannot sell it in the United States.[5]

Although Sheehy is not quite correct that women can't get the natural micronized progesterone, she is speaking to its lack of availability for most women. She then goes on to talk about the intelligent and influential women she spoke to who reacted with disbelief to this quandary. Why, they wondered, should patients and doctors have to use an underground network to obtain a natural product when a government study, supported by their tax dollars, suggests it may be the safest and most effective choice for combined hormone therapy? Sheehy relates her telephone conversation with an FDA administrator, who informed her that no drug company had applied for an application asking to test natural micronized progesterone, and that was the end of the story as far as they were concerned. Sheehy pressed the issue, and in yet another probing conversation with an FDA administrator, she is told that drug companies will now be encouraged to submit applications. In a further conversation, the possibility of an FDA-approved natural progesterone product is estimated as several years down the road.

Sheehy also relates the astonishing fact that the PEPI investigators had to "go out on a limb" to test the natural progesterone in the first place! Imagine: The progestin Provera, with all its known side effects, was somehow the favored drug, and natural progesterone—from which Provera is, in fact, derived—was viewed with suspicion. And when the estrogen/natural progesterone regime is proven to be far superior to the estrogen/progestin regime, women are told that yes, it's *promising*, but in the future.

When Your Doctor Wears Blinders

This is a typical scenario between a midlife woman and her physician:

Nancy's M.D. has put her on Premarin/Provera. Nancy hates taking the Provera. It gives her all sorts of problems—terrible side effects, and she gets her period every month, which she hates. She hears that a friend is using natural progesterone prescribed by her doctor. It works great, says the friend, and yes, she did get her period for a few months but it's now tapered off. And not a single side effect. She even gives Nancy the article in the *New York Times* about the PEPI study that extols the use of oral micronized progesterone. Nancy goes armed with all this information to *her* doctor. He tells her, "Well, I don't know, the natural stuff hasn't been approved by the FDA. Maybe it works, but further tests still need to be done . . ."

And that's the end of that. No prescription for Nancy, a woman who feels she can't move ahead without her doctor's approval. The doctor, on his part, mistakenly believes that because the progesterone is not an FDA approved *drug*, that it is not an FDA approved substance that can be safely prescribed to his patient. The upshot? An even worse situation. Nancy takes the Premarin without the Provera, putting herself at increased risk for uterine cancer.

The Bias Against the Natural

What is the origin of the enormous bias of the medical profession against natural substances? Why have natural substances and herbs been demonized? If you think we're exaggerating, listen to what three women doctors who've written a book on menopause have to say about "natural":

"Estrogen also occurs 'naturally' in some plants. Ginseng contains estrogen and has been promoted as a natural method of treating hot flashes. If this constitutes 'natural' or implied 'safe' treatment, then estrogen derived from pregnant mare's urine (Premarin) should probably be given the same distinction. Seriously, estrogen from any source carries the same risks and benefits and should be taken as a medication in the proper dose and with appropriate medical evaluation and follow-up."[6]

Estrogen "from any source" does *not* carry the same risks and benefits. This is rubbish. They say this because they really don't fully understand herbal medicine, biochemistry, and natural therapeutics, and therefore they devote little more than *one paragraph* in a 367-page book about menopause to making a joke of it. This is the kind of rude dismissal you can frequently hear in the medical profession.

Where does this prejudice come from? Unfortunately, it's what most M.D.'s have been taught in medical school. The way medicine in this country is practiced is primarily to focus on a disease process then treat the symptoms with drugs, frequently without fully addressing the underlying cause. M.D.'s are *drug* oriented; they receive little or no training in natural medicine. When it comes to nutrition, the typical medical student will receive only four to five hours of classes—and these classes are mainly focused on the *negative* aspects of certain foods, such as chocolate aggravating gastric reflux, etc. These students may eventually become doctors who are dedicated, caring, and skilled in many respects, but they will rarely question the origins of their prejudice. And not wanting to seem a little flaky by their peers, they will adopt the standard dismissive attitude toward herbs and the "natural."

At the first Chinese-American Women's Conference in 1990, Dr. Jane Porcino reported that: "Menopause is not an issue in China. Chinese women all exercise, have a low-fat, plant-rich diet, and they take *natural herbs* for discomfort."[7] How many millions of women are we talking about here? And over a period of thousands of years!

Four years later, a conference called "Women and Doctors" was sponsored by Revlon and the UCLA Medical Center. Menopause and its treatment was one of the subjects. At one point, the actress Diane Ladd stood up and demanded to know why there was no nutritionist or natural medicine specialist on the panel. The M.D. chairman of the panel, red-faced and embarrassed, claimed they had wanted a nutritionist but that the conference had been organized very quickly and that no one was available. The organizers later told us that the UCLA doctors had refused to allow any "alternative" practitioners on the panel. They insisted on controlling the debate.

At another point, a questioner asked the panel what dietary recommendations the panel had for breast cancer sufferers. The woman was well-informed and had been reading the masses of new information coming out about the link between diet and breast cancer. The panel members just looked at each other, then suggested she try a low-fat diet.

Later, a female M.D. allowed that she wasn't opposed to a woman trying alternative methods, and that they probably wouldn't hurt. Her tone was: Well, if you think sucking on bark will help you, go ahead, it probably won't kill you. But then she added the caveat: But you should do it under the supervision of your doctor.

The biggest obstacle facing the acceptance of "the naturals" is the established, widespread use of the present HRT treatment. It's now become the 2,000-pound gorilla; it just sits there and you can't move it. So much has been written about HRT that what is repeated often enough takes on the ring of truth. "Factoids" become ingrained in the medical literature and media articles, then are passed from doctor to doctor, patient to patient, etc., making it extremely difficult to weed out the truth.

Then there is the enormous pressure of the drug companies to sell women their drugs and to maintain their control of the market. This is a billion-dollar industry that will fight to maintain the market share of its drugs.

And when it comes to proof of safety and effectiveness, a double standard is applied to natural medicine. From the *New York Times:* "Mainstream medicine can be criticized for overselling its own scientific legitimacy. 'It's reasonable to say that much of existing medicine has not met the standards that alternative medicine is being asked to meet,' says Clyde Behney, an assistant director of the Congressional Office of Technology Assessment."[8]

The Good News

Change is on the way, and it's not a minute too soon. First, the interest in natural medicine among physicians—especially the younger generation—is growing by leaps and bounds. The National Institutes of Health, which recently opened its Office of Alternative Medicine, is funding a study at Columbia University on the influence of diet and plant medicine on women at midlife. Conventional medical schools—including Harvard University, Columbia University, and Washington University—are now teaching nutrition, chiropractic, and acupuncture. And more and more M.D.'s are taking the time to learn about natural medicine, which can lead to greater acceptance of traditional herbal medicine and less reliance on pharmaceutical companies for information on how to treat their patients. And, no small matter, the American public at large is showing a greater interest in remedies outside the boundaries of heavily advertised proprietary products. A new generation of men and women are questioning the very precepts of the "synthetic" drug bias.

And when it comes to treatment for women at midlife, a new generation of women, accustomed to thinking for themselves, is driving the movement toward better, safer, and more effective remedies for hormonal balance. As we've already said, the word is spreading rapidly. The compounding pharmacies testify to the fact that their business in "the naturals" is increasing, in some cases, by up to 400 percent. Scientific backing in the United States is growing for the use of "the naturals," as women do very well on these regimens. These women talk to other women, and they are asking the right questions. Jamie Grifo, M.D., the gynecologist at New York University mentioned earlier, is impressed with the growing support of the scientific literature for "the naturals" and predicts that bio-identical plant-derived hormones will supplant the standard HRT drugs as the most common treatment in less than ten years.

Part Two

THE NATURAL WOMAN PLAN

9

FOLLOWING THE NATURAL WOMAN PLAN

What gets almost entirely lost in current discussions of menopause is why *25 percent* of all American women claim to sail through menopause symptom-free.

Who are these women? What is the difference between them and the women who *do* experience symptoms—ranging from mild to severe—such as hot flashes, night sweats, vaginal dryness, sleeplessness, or thinning hair? Unfortunately, until the recently announced Women's Health Initiative Study, which will not be completed for another ten years, no attempt has been made to amass this kind of information. Western medical science has been the study of why people are ill (disease), not why people are well (wellness).

It seems that women who don't experience symptoms are able somehow to move smoothly through the transition of the cessation of ovulation and menstruation. Their bodies appear to make the adjustment without noticeable disruptions of function. Other women react symptomatically—with differing levels of intensity and duration—to the shifting and diminishing levels of their hormones as they get older.

It is apparent to us that menopause cannot be looked at as an "estrogen deficiency" disease, since the same women who sail through the end of menstruation without incident also experience declines in their measured estrogen levels; yet somehow they can remain asymptomatic and free of "disease." Symptoms, to put it another way, are not *inevitable*.

Eliminating the Word "Menopause"

It would be great to just get rid of the word "menopause" altogether. Too much negativity and fear have accrued to it, and advertising for HRT drugs has compounded the problem by playing to women's fears and insecurities and convincing them that it is a period of inevitable disease. Robert Wilson, M.D., the early salesman for Premarin, contributed greatly to this anxiety by describing menopause in his book *Feminine Forever* as a "mutilation of the whole body," and further intoning that "no woman can be sure of escaping the horror of this living decay."[1]

Such corrosive thinking doesn't belong in the life of the confident women of today. Actually, C. F. Menville, the French physician who first coined the word "menopause" in 1839, struck a much saner note on the subject. Although very much a man of his time, he was able to view in a *positive* way the time period following the end of menstruation. He wrote that, "When the vital forces cease to work together in the interest of the uterus, they go to join those of the mind and the rest of the body. The critical age passed, women have the hope of a longer life than men, their thought acquires more precision, more scope and vitality." He saw his job as mediating the temporary problems that came with this change of function.[2] We view our task in a similar way.

You and Your Hormones

So many factors can play a part in whether a woman will experience physical symptoms related to hormone imbalances. For one thing, menopause, or "The Change," is an event that affects the *mind* and the *body*. How women respond to symptoms is highly individual. Some women can easily shrug off their hot flashes; others will experience them with great sensitivity. Some women can begin to experience symptoms as early as their late thirties. Others will not do so until they reach their fifties. And although the basic monthly menstrual cycle is a given, all women have their unique bodily experiences of it.

To describe a woman's monthly menstrual process in the simplest terms: Estrogen production peaks at ovulation (mid-cycle), at which point progesterone production rises, reaches its peak, and then quickly subsides. If the egg goes unfertilized, the endometrium is sloughed off (i.e., menstrual bleeding), and then the cycle begins again. Two other hormones produced in the pituitary gland in the brain, LH (luteinizing hormone) and FSH (follicle stimulating hormone), play their part as "signaling" mechanisms for the process.

The biochemical process that choreographs these functions is more complex. It begins in the brain when the hypothalamus sends a chemical message to the pituitary gland to release the hormones LH and FSH. At first, FSH is sent out in a greater amount, which stimulates the ovaries to develop and enlarge several follicles (human egg cells). At this point, estrogen recruited by LH causes the lining of the uterus to grow, in preparation for implantation of an embryo. After about fourteen days, the hypothalamus orders the slowing down of FSH production and the stepping up of LH production. This causes the ovary to release the growing egg (ovulation). The ruptured follicles left behind when the egg escapes are called the corpus luteum (yellow body), from which is produced progesterone. The time from ovulation to just before menstruation is called the luteal phase, during which blood vessels and connective tissues in the endometrium, or lining of the uterus, proliferate and enlarge, readying the uterus for implantation of a fertilized egg. If the egg isn't fertilized, the corpus luteum will stop producing hormones, bringing on the shedding of the blood-rich uterine lining and signaling the restarting of menstruation.

As a woman gets older and fewer egg follicles are stimulated, the amount of estrogen and progesterone produced declines. Menstruation then becomes scantier and often erratic, eventually subsiding. On average, from approximately the ages of forty-five to fifty-two, a woman begins to experience wide fluctuations in her hormone levels. This can cause hormone excesses and/or deficiencies, as well as an alteration of the ratios not only between estrogen and progesterone, but between other important regulating hormones as well, resulting in any number of symptoms, the primary ones being: *hot flashes*, which are feelings of extreme heat that may last as long as five minutes; and *vaginal dryness and thinning*, wherein the vaginal walls become thinner as estrogen levels drop. Other symptoms include *loss of libido, depression, mood swings, memory loss, headaches, loss of concentration, erratic mood changes, a feeling of being on pins and needles, fatigue,* and *forgetfulness.* These symptoms can occur at varying times, and for varying durations and intensities over as long a period as ten to fifteen years. (See appendix G for a complete list of symptoms that can be attributed to menopausal changes.)

What Triggers Hormonal Imbalance Symptoms?

By the time they become aware of midlife changes in their bodies, most Western women would benefit from some kind of support against hormonal imbalances. And for the U.S. women who've had hysterectomies, hormone replacement becomes a *necessity,* because even if the ovaries are not removed, the woman's ability to produce hormones naturally is interrupted. Many different factors can contribute to a woman becoming symptomatic, but Western women seem to be experiencing earlier and earlier menopauses, and more are manifesting symptoms. This means that there are a growing number of pressure points in a Western woman's life that affect her hormonal balance. The primary ones appear to be genetics, stress, anovulatory cycles (that is, menstruation without ovulation, see below), PMS, the use of birth control pills, premature menopause, surgical menopause, diet, lack of exercise, and the impact of the environment. You need to understand each of these to appreciate how the Natural Woman plan works.

Genetics. Here the old-fashioned but apt word "constitution" comes into play: Some women are of the more hearty type; hormonal fluctuations don't seem to register on their body screens. They sail easily through the storms. On the other end of the spectrum are the women who are vastly more sensitive—every change is exquisitely felt and is manifested as a symptom. Some women are just born with hormone levels that are genetically more stable.

Stress. Chronic stress over long periods of time can lead to nutritional as well as adrenal gland depletion, which sets you up for the symptoms of hormonal imbalance. Other organs in the body, primarily the adrenal glands, are programmed to take over from the ovaries when their hormone production declines, but if you've overtaxed your adrenals, they won't be able to do their job when you need them.

Anovulatory cycles. Recent studies have shown that increasing numbers of women are having anovulatory cycles beginning as early as their mid-thirties; *that is, they menstruate, but they do not ovulate.* Peter Ellison, Ph.D., of Harvard University, has done a number of studies that show this alarming trend.[3] In Canada, Jerilynn Prior, M.D., a professor of endocrinology at the University of British Columbia, found when studying women—particularly athletes—that anovulatory cycles were very common. Some athletes who trained very hard stopped menstruating altogether.[4]

Unless you're monitoring your own cycles—if you are infertile and trying to get pregnant, for example—you would not be aware of this lack of ovulation. But the effect on your hormonal world is significant: If you're not ovulating, then you don't produce progesterone during the ovulation cycle, which means that your body is producing a lower amount of progesterone overall, which signifies that estrogen is in at least relative excess in your body, leaving you vulnerable to hormonal imbalance symptoms, including osteoporosis, as the role of progesterone in bone building is just beginning to be recognized.

Besides anovulation, the causes of progesterone deficiency can be varied. The use of progestins can interfere with the body's natural production of progesterone. It has been suggested that *progesterone depletion* in both men and women is a growing problem in our society, that the pressure of toxins in the environment leads to this condition. Physical stress on the body can also be a significant factor, but more alarmingly, the reasons for this growing phenomenon may still be unknown. This condition can trigger a rise in PMS symptoms in women, as their bodies will be dealing with an imbalance between estrogen and progesterone due to a lack of progesterone production; of even greater concern, progesterone depletion can also account for the growing rise in infertility in women.[5]

PMS. If you've experienced PMS to a significant degree, you have suffered through some of the effects of hormonal imbalance and, in all likelihood, you will manifest menopausal symptoms to some degree. It has been only twenty years since the idea of PMS has become accepted as a medically valid syndrome, but even now, it is not always understood or treated by most doctors as a manifestation of hormonal imbalance. It is often treated with pain medication, diuretics, or antidepressants. All these remedies are prescribed to treat the symptoms of PMS, but none of them recognize or treat the underlying cause.

Consider the case of postpartum syndrome: New mothers can experience severe depression after giving birth, but only in the last few years has it been acknowledged that low progesterone levels are the likely culprit. Now women suffering from postpartum syndrome are being treated with progesterone, with great effectiveness. In fact, the whole notion of hormone balance as the key to both emotional and physical health in women has been slow to penetrate Western medicine.

Birth control pill use. The effect of using birth control pills on a woman's subsequent menopausal period is in large measure an unstudied phenomenon, but birth control pills—which work by suppressing your native hormones—can themselves lead to many health problems. Many of the problems of estrogen dominance, including fluid retention, depression, headaches, and urinary tract infections, are experienced by women using birth control pills. Everything we've said about the negative effects for menopausal women of using progestins applies to the progestins used in birth control pills. Having altered your normal hormonal cycles when using the Pill, you are more prone to symptoms at midlife as well as potentially more serious health problems. This is because the synthetic estrogens and progestins used in the Pill can interfere with the body's own progesterone receptors. The progestins are more potent and may inhibit the production of your body's own sex hormones.

Premature menopause. For a growing number of women in their mid-thirties, the combination of stress, inadequate nutritional intake, anovulatory cycles, adrenal insufficiency, birth control pill use, and other factors can lead to a number of problems, including fibrocystic breasts and uterine fibroids. These women are too young to be considered as being in "The Change," as their periods are continuing, but they are not feeling very well at all. This is a time when these women are in the greatest danger of getting hysterectomized—harking back to the old practice of "just cut out the offending organ" when a woman becomes too emotional.

Surgical menopause. It should be shocking to learn that one-third of all women in the United States have had hysterectomies, and that in the age sixty bracket the number increases to one-half. It is further estimated that the average age for this operation is thirty-five.[6] Hidden within these statistics is the fact that in many medical quarters—principally among those who profit from the operation—the aftereffects of this operation on a woman's body and on her subsequent health are not taken seriously enough. The ramifications in terms of the body can be global. Some of the immediate symptoms can include loss of hair, headaches, palpitations, and loss of sex drive. Forty percent of hysterectomized women can suffer severe depression, not to mention the amount of suffering that goes unreported.[7]

All women who have had this hormonal disruption are going to experience fallout from it in the form of symptoms—some immediate and very obvious, some less so—since they have undergone a dramatic interference with their hormonal control system, resulting from a sudden sharp drop in estrogen, progesterone, and testosterone production. Even those women who had only their uteruses removed, leaving the ovaries, *will* have some disruption in hormonal function. Progesterone levels frequently fall within several months of the operation, and estrogen levels may fall within a year or two. For the woman who has had both a hysterectomy *and* her ovaries removed, hormone replenishment is a necessity at least for the first few years after the operation. At a later time, once they have replenished and balanced their hormone levels, many of these women can shift to a maintenance program. This will be described in more detail in chapter 10.

Diet. Before the age of thirty-five, it's possible to sail through life on a poor diet, but after thirty-five, you will in all likelihood start paying the price in the form of an overall decrease in energy and health, with a general susceptibility to hormonal imbalance symptoms. As with the effect of stress, if your nutritional status is low, then your body starts to tap into other backup systems, which you will pay for in the form of hormonal fluctuation, leading inevitably to symptoms.

Lack of exercise. An overly sedentary lifestyle can affect your hormonal balance and have an impact on your overall health, which, in turn, affects your hormonal balance, getting you into a negative health spiral.

Environment. We are all more or less at the mercy of pollution, pesticides, and all the other environmental horrors that can have an impact on our health. Both men and women can experience the effect of *xenoestrogens*—those foreign estrogenic substances that can mimic and/or interfere with your body's own hormones—in the form of infertility, hormonal imbalances, birth defects, decreased libido, and cancers and other diseases. Xenoestrogens are principally found in the petrochemicals that proliferate in our environment. They are part of a larger category of chemicals referred to as *xenobiotics*, but since the majority of these mimic estrogen, the more frequently used term is xenoestrogen. Here is where all women (and men) need support. There is growing evidence of the rise in breast cancer in areas where there has been a large use of pesticides, which is why all women, no matter how well they feel, should fortify themselves by using diet and supplements to strengthen the immune system against attack, minimize damage, and expedite toxin elimination.

The Natural Woman Plan: Overall Balancing for Total Well-Being

Our goal is for *all* women to sail through menopause and live a long, healthy life using a combination of diet, exercise, nutritional supplementation, and hormone balancing as needed. The Natural Woman plan aims to not only help you mediate the temporary problems and changes of midlife, but to go beyond that and learn to use natural resources in order to maximize the potential for health, beauty, and vitality over the long term.

The plan we are presenting is one for overall balancing, featuring treatment protocols for the underlying problem, not just individual symptoms. Not *this* for hot flashes, *that* for palpitations, *this* for headaches, *that* for night sweats, *this* for depression and agitation, *that* for loss of sexual libido, and so on. There are, for example, differences of opinion about which of a woman's hormones is most responsible for her sexual vitality, and therefore confusion over how to best treat it, as well as a great risk of misdiagnosis. However, by following the principle of overall hormone balancing, including dietary changes and exercise, and by looking at the whole woman and not just one complaint, a woman's sexual vitality can be restored or even increased naturally.

Every woman will experience hormonal shifts in her own unique way, but no matter who you are, if you address the fundamental issues of hormone balancing, the symptoms will be mitigated. Symptoms are signs of imbalance—a symptom is not the imbalance itself. Our goal is to correct the underlying imbalance, thereby automatically relieving the symptom. In a way similar to what women have done for thousands of years, we will be using the miraculous power of plants to help us sail through the rough seas.

We are also firm believers in preventive measures. There are a growing number of doctors who believe that by recognizing hormonal imbalance factors early, the onset of negative symptoms for American women at menopause can be virtually eliminated. By taking an interest in your hormone levels *before* you become symptomatic, and then monitoring those hormone levels and slowly adding your unique hormone replenishment mixture as needed, the onset of negative symptoms can be avoided.

Can I Regulate Menopausal Symptoms with Just Dietary Changes?

Absolutely. But by the time most women begin to be symptomatic, they are almost certainly, to some degree, in nutritional and hormonal "deficit." They often need extra help in mediating their hormonal shiftings and frequently some temporary intervention with herbal formulas or plant-derived hormone replenishment. A large number of women can completely control menopausal symptoms through diet, supplements, and lifestyle changes without additional hormonal support. Those women who need hormonal assistance in the beginning in many cases can move off hormone replenishment after a period of six months to a few years and do just fine with the Natural Woman dietary and supplement and exercise plan. If needed, a woman can then use "the naturals" on occasion in times of increased need. Her personal experience will dictate the protocol.

The key to the Natural Woman plan is its focus on all the contributing factors to a woman's overall wellness, and therefore simply taking "the naturals" without making a change in diet or exercise habits simply won't reap the same benefits, such as overall well-being, vitality, sexual energy, and attractiveness. If you take "the naturals" for symptoms, but then continue on a way of life that includes overindulgence in alcohol, caffeine, and fatty foods, you're going to be working against the effectiveness of "the naturals" and you will not be protecting your body sufficiently against the effects of aging.

It's certainly easier to swallow a pill than to begin to eat vegetables regularly and start an exercise regime. But the benefit of following our plan is nothing less than a long, healthy life. A pill may help you deal with temporary symptoms but it can only do so much in protecting you from today's biggest killers, the chronic degenerative diseases like heart disease, osteoporosis, and cancer.

Fortunately, the generation of women now reaching their forties is more accustomed to exercising in gyms, paying attention to their diets, and looking to the natural in all areas of their lives; they are also more likely to see the importance of adding these factors to their daily routines.

Keeping It Simple

How hormones work in the body is vastly complex, but when it comes to regulating them, the guiding principle is to keep it simple and keep it bio-identical. When it comes to hormone balancing, *less* can definitely be *more.* Taking more hormone replenishment than you need will not make you more youthful. Again, balance is the key. There is always an "optimum" hormone dosage. Think of the level used in carpentry: It registers when a piece of wood is in exact balance, and so it is with hormone dosage. This book will help you do just that by guiding you to bio-identical hormone products that match your own hormones exactly. In addition, it will show you how to get the benefit of the natural plant-based diet that has shown its effectiveness for women for thousands of years. Following this program will help you continue to be the best you can be.

10

HOW TO USE "THE NATURALS"

Although we look forward to a day when the standard definitions used in "medical menopause" can be done away with, we will be using them here for overall convenience. Our ultimate goal is for women to glide through the cessation of menstruation by, from an early age, staying in tune with their bodies, eating right, and exercising, then replenishing and balancing hormones if needed.

We don't claim that our plan is the only way to replenish hormones, just a *better* way than the standard HRT drugs. The Natural Woman plan takes you off potentially dangerous or imbalanced drugs, utilizing, when necessary, plant-derived bio-identical hormone products that are without the side effects and risk factors associated with conventional HRT drugs. There are many other effective natural remedies that can also work quite well to relieve hormonal imbalance symptoms, and although they are outside our focus here, in appendix D we will give a brief description of some key herbs that can be used singly or in combination in the treatment of menopausal symptoms. These herbs are also found in some of the herbal products we are recommending as part of the plan. They can be the sole primary treatment for many women; for other women they work well as a complementary treatment to "the naturals."

In this chapter, we will be providing a "boilerplate" treatment that can be adjusted for your individual needs. As every woman comes with her unique biochemistry and medical and lifestyle history, you must work with your doctor to determine the exact dose that is right for you. A dose that works for one woman may be too strong or too weak for another. Also remember that we are presenting a *complete* plan. To get the full benefit of "the naturals," and to come out of this passage healthier, more fit, and more beautiful than before, "the naturals" should be taken in conjunction with the diet, exercise, and supplement recommendations.

Working with Your Doctor

If you already have a doctor you are comfortable with, tell him/her you want to try this plan for six months. If he is unfamiliar with "the naturals," or resistant to the idea, have him call (or call yourself) a compounding pharmacy that specializes in this treatment (see appendix). In many areas of the U.S., nurse practitioners can provide guidance and facilitate prescriptions. Several of the large compounders with extensive mail-order businesses, such as Women's International Pharmacy, Bajamar, Madison, and Apothecure, have 800 numbers and are very experienced with dealing with doctors. They have compelling scientific research and educational material for informing you and your doctor.

If you are not getting the cooperation you want from your physician, you must make a decision about getting a second opinion or referral. If you need a referral for a second opinion or don't have a doctor, there are several ways to go about finding a doctor who can work with you in using "the naturals." The Natural Woman Institute is accumulating a database of doctors adept in the use of "the naturals" and will provide you with the best available information (see appendix A for details). Other organizations, such as the American College for the Advancement of Medicine, that are not affiliated with either the compounding pharmacies or the large pharmaceutical houses, can be excellent sources of information. In addition, the compounding pharmacists who specialize in "the naturals" maintain lists of doctors who use their services and can mail these lists to you. The International Academy of Compounding Pharmacists can direct you to a pharmacist near you, who, in turn, can provide you with names of doctors they work with in your area.

As we've said, finding the right doctor may not be an easy task for all women, but over the next few years, we expect this situation to change dramatically. In the meantime, a woman must do her part in pursuing treatment and learning all she can.

If you are already taking Premarin/Provera or other HRT drugs, a compounding pharmacist can work up an equivalent dose of "the naturals." Switching is almost never a problem. Usually, if a woman is having trouble with her Premarin/Provera regimen, she will often experience great relief and satisfaction almost immediately, or within a few days, after switching to "the naturals."

Testing

The area of hormonal testing is still evolving, and tests can be interpreted differently by different physicians. However, getting a battery of tests will allow you to at least monitor your own levels to arrive at a starting point for effective treatment. Many internists and gynecologists put women on the HRT drugs without testing their hormone levels. Some just test a woman's LH and FSH levels. Although we recommend getting full testing of all hormone levels—a full steroid panel, as it's called—if your doctor is unable to interpret the results, it won't be that helpful, and the best measure will be how you feel.

Jesse Hanley, M.D., a Malibu, California, family physician with ten years' experience in using "the naturals," recommends getting a complete panel of blood-serum levels of at least total estrogens (E1, E2, E3) and progesterone, depending on how much testing a woman can afford. A more complete panel would include testosterone and DHEA, thyroid and liver functions. In her experience, just testing LH and FSH levels can give highly fluctuating results. A woman's LH and FSH levels can be elevated in one test, showing that she is menopausal, then, six months later, be back to the levels of a premenopausal woman. Dr. Hanley's experience with testing is corroborated by Dr. Christiane Northrup, the author of *Women's Bodies, Women's Wisdom,* who has also advocated and prescribed "the naturals" for over ten years.

Uzzi Reiss, M.D., an obstetrician/gynecologist trained both in Israel and the United States, and whose Beverly Hills practice has been a pioneer in the use of "the naturals," emphasizes that what is for one woman a normal level can be quite different for another. In addition, a woman taking *x* amount of estrogen will experience a *y* rise in levels, but for another the same amount of estrogen can cause a greater or lesser rise. For Dr. Reiss, the key is individualized treatment and resolve on the part of the physician to pay close attention to how the patient is responding and to her overall feeling of well-being.

In addition to the standard blood tests and 24-hour urine testing, two new tests have recently been added to the arsenal, bringing more convenience and accuracy to the process, which you should bring to your doctor's attention if he or she is unfamiliar with them.

Salivary hormonal analysis. You no longer need to drive to the doctor's office to get a measurement of your hormone levels (the steroid panel of tests). You can send a saliva sample test from your home to Aeron Laboratories (see appendix C). You do not need a prescription and can order this test for yourself. Your saliva hormone profile gives an index of what are known as "free" hormone levels in the blood (not bound to protein). This test is easy, affordable, accurate, and painless, and could shortly replace the standard blood test. Your doctor may not be aware of it, but you should make a point of asking for it and/or sending away for information yourself.

Osteoporosis risk assay. Every woman over forty should monitor her bone density. Monitoring your bone health and integrity has become easier and much safer. Instead of having to expose yourself to follow-up X rays after you've had a baseline X ray, you can take a twenty-four-hour urine test called NTx Bone Loss Assay. It measures your bone loss by using a biological marker called Type I collagen. You can use this test to adjust your hormone replenishment program. It's simple and affordable. (See appendix C for resources and other osteoporosis test information.)

Interpreting the Tests

A practical follow-up plan has been proposed by Madison Pharmacy in conjunction with Aeron labs. Marla Ahlgrimm, R.Ph., the founder of Madison Pharmacy, one of the first pharmacies in this country to specialize in "the naturals," offers a consultation service for both physicians and patients on test interpretation. This program proposes an initial panel of saliva tests, followed by a prescription. In thirty days, another saliva test is collected to analyze the absorption and adequacy of the prescribed treatment. Dosages can then be adjusted. In six months, another saliva test and a urine test are used to measure the effect of the prescription on bone. Finally, a woman can be placed on a yearly maintenance evaluation to keep watch on her progress.

Is Testing Absolutely Necessary for Every Woman?

After listening to her accounting of her symptoms, and taking a good history of a woman's medical and menstrual background, it may be appropriate for your doctor to prescribe "the naturals" with adjusted diet, supplements, and exercise as the primary prescription without first testing hormone levels. But after six months, it is a prudent and reasonable medical expenditure to test the woman to make sure the protocol is working for her: Are her hormone levels acceptable? Has her osteoporosis risk gone down? Also, if the initial prescription is not completely effective, testing is an important way to uncover whether there is uniqueness in the woman's hormonal makeup and to help come up with an alternative program.

Choosing the Form of "The Naturals" That's Right for You

Basically, there are two sources for "the naturals": compounded products ordered from the compounding pharmacists, for which you will always need a doctor's prescription, and commercial preformulated products, some of which can be obtained over the counter.

Over-the-Counter Products

There are a number of progesterone creams sold over the counter. If we had to give an award for pioneering achievement in the breakthrough of "the naturals" in this country, it would certainly go to Pro-Gest®. A suspension of natural progesterone in vitamin E oil, this cream was developed by the biologist Raymond Peat, Ph.D., along with Bruce MacFarland, Ph.D. At a speech at the California Orthomolecular Society in 1978, Peat presented a paper on natural progesterone for use with PMS. John Lee, M.D., a California family physician who attended the meeting, was very impressed with the presentation and then began using progesterone with his menopausal patients. Following his great success with the product, Lee would go on to become one of the leading proponents of the use of progesterone for the prevention and reversal of osteoporosis.

Pro-Gest® is a genuine grassroots success story: Word of its effectiveness and superiority over progestins for both PMS and menopausal symptoms was passed from woman to woman. Its effectiveness also established the use of a transdermal (absorbed through the skin) cream as an effective and safe delivery system for progesterone. The company now sells 10,000 jars a month.

However, beware of so-called wild yam creams that are proliferating on the shelves of health food stores. There is a misconception that wild yam and the bio-identical hormones *synthesized* from wild yam are the same and have the same effect.

In studies that were done to test the hormonal activity of certain wild yam products, it was shown that only creams that contained added bio-identical hormones showed significant hormone receptor activity. Pro-Gest, one of those that tested high in stimulating hormone receptor activity, has been in use for over twenty years, and Dr. Laux has used it with hundreds of patients with a very high level of success. In our protocols we will be using Pro-Gest as the recommended progesterone replenishment product (see appendix C for a complete list of potencies of other progesterone preparations).

The advantage of the compounded products in comparison to the over-the-counter products is that they can be designed specifically for you, and don't contain unwanted additives. In addition, if you are a woman who needs to supplement estrogen as well as progesterone, then you will need to work with the compounding pharmacies.

Herbal Products

Remifemin, distributed in the U.S. by Enzymatic Therapy, is a standardized herbal extract of the herb black cohosh (*Cimicifuga racemosa),* which we will be recommending as part of our treatment plan. It is newly available in the United States as a dietary supplement. Developed in Germany by Schaper & Bruemmer, we single it out because it has been extensively used and tested in Europe for over forty years and has been proven to be very safe and effective. No other herbal commercial product has an equivalent track record. It is the number one best-selling product for menopause and PMS in Germany. Remifemin can be used by women in any category, but particularly for women in perimenopause or menopause with mild symptoms, it is a good option. Black cohosh is an herb that contains compounds that exert estrogenic effects. They behave in a similar fashion to human estriol and exert a balancing action on your native estrogen; if your estrogen levels are low, they enhance the estrogen effects; if estrogen levels are high, they reduce the estrogen effects.[1]

Remifemin can be used safely by women with breast cancer or women who are at high risk, as it doesn't stimulate cell growth in the breast.

There are several other effective herbal packaged products on the market, such as MENO-FEM from Prevail and Vitanica Women's Phase II, which contain traditional herbal medicines that have brought relief to menopausal women for centuries and can be used as well. MENO-FEM, which is doctor formulated and sold widely in North America, contains gamma oryzanol, a rice bran oil extract. This substance has been studied extensively in Japan, and has shown proven results for menopausal symptoms. Dr. Laux has used it with significant success. The formula also contains plant enzymes to make it more digestible and absorbable. Vitanica Women's Phase I and II is an herbal formula designed by Dr. Tori Hudson, a naturopathic physician who specializes in menopausal treatment. The formula contains well-known herbs traditionally used for menopausal symptoms; these herbs have been tested effectively in clinical studies run by Dr. Hudson.

These herbal formulas have the benefit of being natural, inexpensive, and readily available without prescription. For those women who either can't afford the prescription "naturals" or would prefer these herbal choices, they represent an excellent choice. They cover a broad spectrum of discomforts and can be used for many women as primary intervention, along with diet, exercise, and supplementation. Women with more severe or intractable symptoms and/or surgical menopause frequently will need to use the prescription "naturals."

Delivery Systems

When it comes to using "the naturals," you have a lot of options. The compounding pharmacists can prepare hormones in a variety of delivery systems, from creams, gels, and drops to oral tablets or suppositories. What you choose to use is based on your preference, and, in some instances, how your body responds.

Some women love using the creams, others find them messy. European companies frequently prepare "the naturals" in gel form with handy applicators that allow you to measure out an exact dose, and this formulation is gaining some acceptance in this country. The transdermal (absorbed through the skin) creams and gels are applied to those parts of your body where the skin is thin and the cream can be easily absorbed—e.g., inner wrists, inner arms, face, stomach, breasts, neck, and palms of the hands, all the places where capillaries are abundant and close to the surface (where you blush). They can work when rubbed on the stomach as well. Some doctors prefer to prescribe "the naturals" as oral drops as they believe women can regulate their dosages more easily in this way. Some women insist on oral tablets, and many doctors prefer prescribing them for the simple reason that they have a long familiarity with prescribing in this form.

The transdermal creams and gels have the great advantage of delivering the hormone directly into your bloodstream, where it is carried through your body. In this form, the hormones bypass the liver's first-pass removal process, allowing greater immediate systemic effect. Women with gastrointestinal problems or liver problems are advised to use the transdermals.

If you decide to take "the naturals" orally, the product as prepared by a compounding pharmacist will have been *micronized.* A micronized hormone product is one that has been broken down into very small particles and suspended in an oil base, then "compounded" into capsules or slow-release tablets. It is absorbed through the lymph system and goes directly into circulation, thereby avoiding the digestive tract and decreasing the liver's first-pass removal.[2] One of the liver's primary jobs is to break down and render harmless unneeded hormones, protecting you from imbalances and overstimulation of tissues. Your liver will prevent much of the hormone from going into circulation by breaking it down. This removal of the hormones by your liver reduces the effective dose that you are taking and can produce liver damage, one of the side effects of traditional HRT.

Another very common delivery system is the patch, but many women hate the idea of having something stuck to their bottom all the time. It can also be irritating to the skin, and its adhesive backing contains undesirable chemicals. In any case, we only recommend using plant-derived estradiol (E2) (the only form in which patches now come), balanced by progesterone, for women who have just begun surgical menopause, or women who have symptoms that are nonresponsive to the tri-est formula.

Overall, we prefer the transdermals, because of their better ability to maintain blood-hormone levels with smaller doses without the risks of the larger oral doses. Because of our unique biochemical individuality, some women may need to experiment to discover which form gives them the greatest results and continuing effectiveness.

How to Make "The Naturals" Work for You

We have broken down the use of "the naturals" into five general categories of symptoms: premature menopause/PMS, peri-menopause, surgical menopause, menopause, and post-menopause. As a general rule of thumb, you should look to the lowest dose and the simplest treatment first. In terms of efficacy, cost, and intervention, less is better. In almost all cases, choosing the lowest possible dose and the simplest approach is the best. The dosages listed are a guide for women and their doctors. If a woman is already using Premarin or other HRT drugs, she should work with her doctor. The protocols are designed to aid both the woman and her doctor, and if you choose to go with the compounded products you will need a prescription.

Pay Attention to How You Feel

This may seem obvious, but you'd be amazed at how often women are simply not in touch with what is going on in their bodies. Given the lack of unanimity about test interpretation, it is all the more important that you tune in to your own signals. There are doctors who take the position that once they've supplied the "estrogen," the woman just has to live with any "inconvenient" side effects that come with it. But every woman is different. A dose that works perfectly for a friend might be a little off for you and will need to be adjusted. Use your own judgment. Overall well-being is a key factor in determining the right choices for yourself.

PMS and Premature Menopause

The number of women suffering from these conditions seems to be increasing and is clearly influenced by excess stress, poor diet, environmental factors, and drug use, including taking birth control pills. Women in what we are calling pre-menopause—early to late thirties to early forties—can have generally regular periods but still suffer from symptoms associated with menopause.

In the case of PMS, many of the symptoms associated with it (such as bloating, headaches, anxiety, etc.) are the same as what is labeled for older women close to the cessation of menstruation "estrogen dominance." PMS is now a recognized syndrome, but it is by no means an *inevitable* syndrome for young women. What has been slow to enter conventional medical practice is the understanding that PMS is at a fundamental level a function of hormonal imbalance and can be positively averted with proper diet, exercise, and the temporary use of natural progesterone. This therapy, pioneered in Europe by Dr. Katharina Dalton, has been successfully in use in this country since the early eighties. Those women who would like to help themselves (or their young daughters) and want even more information about PMS should get a copy of Dr. Dalton's book, *Once a Month.*[3]

BASIC PROTOCOL

PMS

We recommend using a progesterone cream, either Pro-Gest® or a preparation prepared by a compounding pharmacy, but those who prefer it can take oral micronized progesterone. The most common prescription is 25 to 100 milligrams twice daily.

The recommended Pro-Gest® regime is as follows:

Starting on day 14 of your menstrual cycle (or the day after ovulation if you know it), apply ⅛ teaspoon of cream on days 14 to 17, then ¼ teaspoon on days 18 to 22, then ½ teaspoon of progesterone cream until the start of the menses, and then stop. Start again next month at the same time. You can use a kitchen measuring spoon as an applicator to get your accurate dosage. Alternate application of the cream on your wrists, inner arms, stomach, thighs, or neck. After three, and usually within six, months of regular use you will notice that your symptoms are less pronounced.

You can then start your progesterone treatment when your first symptoms come at any time in the month. Usually, by this time they are less severe and less frequent, if not completely gone. If symptoms disappear completely, stop treatment and use again if they return.

Premature Menopause

The number of women who actually stop having their periods before forty has been estimated at approximately 8 percent.[4] A common practice is to treat symptomatic women with birth control pills, which means that they are being given a *progestin* to control symptoms. Although the progestin can alleviate symptoms, using natural progesterone is preferable and more beneficial for all the reasons we have already stated.

Remifemin: 1 tablet, 2 times daily. You may experience relief from symptoms quickly, but therapeutic effects will be better evaluated after four weeks of treatment and thereafter; the longer the duration of treatment the greater the rate of improvement. MENO-FEM from Prevail and Vitanica Women's Phase I are also good choices.

and/or

Progesterone: Same as PMS protocol above.

Remifemin or other herbal products can frequently alleviate PMS symptoms. Given time, the herbal products combined with supplements are often sufficient, and progesterone can be added during times of added stress. Because the herbal regime takes effect more slowly, those women who want relief more quickly can turn directly to the natural progesterone.

Peri-Menopause—or, the Forgotten Woman

The period of so-called peri-menopause—for the average woman the age range is forty-five to forty-nine—is usually described as a time when a woman's estrogen levels can fluctuate wildly. These women can experience the same symptoms as menopausal women, but they are still menstruating. Dr. Jamie Grifo of New York University says that, unfortunately, these women are frequently treated like orphans who can't find a proper home anywhere and that more attention should be paid to their overall well-being.[5] The focus on whether or not to replace *estrogen* as the sole criteria for treatment creates a blindness to other factors causing "menopausal" symptoms, and because standard practitioners don't usually have herbal remedies and tonics in their cabinets, the peri-menopausal woman frequently slips through the cracks of standard treatment.

The case of Ellen D. is typical. In her mid-forties and still menstruating, she was having very distressing symptoms: sudden weight gain, mood swings, *zero* interest in sex, occasional hot flashes, insomnia, and depression. Her doctor measured her estrogen levels—which were deemed "normal"—and declared it "too soon" for HRT. However, this peri-menopause period is one of so-called estrogen dominance, when a woman's body may be producing smaller amounts of progesterone in relation to her estrogen. Ellen's doctor didn't check her progesterone levels, or look for an underlying cause for the symptoms. He just sent her home and told her to live with it. She is just "that age."

So Ellen tried to help herself the best she could. She dieted strenuously to combat the weight gain, which didn't go away. She took sleeping pills for the insomnia. Still, she felt awful. Her frustrating search went on for several years; it was only when she began to use a progesterone cream under Dr. Laux's care that she was able to deal with what were symptoms of estrogen dominance—wild fluctuations of estrogen in relation to unbalanced progesterone levels.

Another way the peri-menopause woman can get inappropriate treatment is when a doctor *does* prescribe estrogen unnecessarily during this phase. Dr. Jesse Hanley recounts that she sees numerous women who come to her after having been given estrogen and reacting badly. Adding estrogen for these women can only further complicate the symptoms of "estrogen dominance." She treats these women with progesterone and they do very well. The progesterone can balance the estrogen's effect. And, as a precursor hormone, progesterone can convert to estrogen in a woman's body over time, if there is a need for it. For the peri-menopausal woman this can definitely be the best first line of treatment.

BASIC PROTOCOL

Remifemin, MENO-FEM, or Vitanica Phase II: As directed.
and/or

Progesterone: *25 to 200 milligrams daily in divided doses* (oral). If you wish to use a cream, the compounding pharmacist will make up an equivalent dose. If your symptoms are intense, you can take this dose continuously throughout the month. After 1 to 3 months most women feel more hormonally stable; we then suggest taking your progesterone cyclically for 12 days, starting at what would be the middle of your normal cycle. You can stay with your continuous progesterone treatment if your symptoms dictate this, but we usually recommend a cyclic approach that mimics your body's wisdom once your system and symptoms are stabilized. Another good choice is Pro-Gest® cream, as directed on package. If your symptoms aren't alleviated with just progesterone therapy, or you know through lab tests that estrogen is needed, then we suggest:

Tri-est and progesterone: *1.25 to 2.50 milligrams total estrogen.* A dose of ½ teaspoon of tri-est cream plus progesterone equals 2 milligrams of total estrogen (1.6 milligrams estriol, 0.2 milligram estrone, 0.2 milligram estradiol) and 25 to 100 milligrams of progesterone. Apply this dose twice daily, morning and evening, throughout the month. Again, you can use this for twenty-five days on and five days off, or you may use it continuously, straight through the month. If your symptoms allow, and you can follow this schedule, we recommend taking the five days off. However, this combination of "the naturals" does not in general cause significant stimulation of uterine tissue proliferation and, therefore, there is no need to stop due to induced menstruation and the tissue sloughing common to conventional HRT therapy. (Some physicians prefer a bi-estrogen product, which is 20% estradiol and 80% estriol. Although we are using tri-est as the standard prescription, preliminary reports indicate that bi-estrogen is effective.)

Surgical Menopause

If you have had your uterus and your ovaries removed in what is frequently termed a "complete hysterectomy," then it is very important for you to get a full steroid panel of tests. Your ovaries make more than just estrogen. You want to measure the levels of all your sex hormones—estrogen and progesterone, plus testosterone and DHEA. These hormones have effects throughout your entire body, including your brain. Once considered a hormone from which other hormones were made and of little value in and of itself, an understanding of the importance of DHEA to the aging process and other bodily functions is growing. Women interested in its functions should consult recent books on the subject, including *The Super-Hormone Promise* by William Regelson, M.D., and Carol Colman.

While any menopausal woman may benefit from this more complete hormonal balancing, it is particularly important for women who have been hysterectomized and have, therefore, experienced a severe assault on their bodies and their hormonal systems. A thorough hormone replenishment program of more than just estrogen and progesterone can improve their energy, memory, sex drive, and overall immunity.

If you are a woman who has been prescribed only Premarin because your doctor said you did not need progesterone, since you no longer have a uterus, we disagree. Typically—as happened in Chris's case—a woman is handed a prescription for Premarin and told to continue it for the rest of her life. Whatever unpleasant symptoms are experienced—such as extreme weight gain for some women—are chalked up to unfortunate but unavoidable side effects. Not only do we recommend that you switch to a bio-identical estrogen product, but we also recommend that you add natural progesterone, which has protective and balancing effects throughout your body. For example, use of natural progesterone can limit water retention and weight gain, enhance the functions of your central nervous system, and help protect your breasts from cell changes that can lead to cancer, and unlike Provera has been shown to protect against vasospasms of coronary arteries.

To all other women reading this book, avoid hysterectomy. With everything we now know about the importance of a woman's uterus and ovaries to her overall health, it is clear that the removal of these organs should only be a last resort. Many good books have already been written on this subject, including *The Hysterectomy Hoax,* by Stanley West, M.D., who has stated flatly that hysterectomy is almost never necessary except when a woman has cancer. Another book on the subject is *No More Hysterectomies,* by Vicki Hufnagel, M.D.

BASIC PROTOCOL

Estradiol and progesterone (oral): *0.5 milligram E2/25 to 100 milligrams progesterone two times a day, morning and evening.* After approximately one year, you can gradually move to a tri-est and progesterone formula.

Tri-est and progesterone: *1.5 to 2.50 milligrams total estrogen.* A dose of ½ teaspoon of tri-est cream plus progesterone equals 2 milligrams total estrogen (1.6 milligrams estriol, 0.2 milligram estrone, 0.2 milligram estradiol) and 25 to 100 milligrams progesterone. Apply this dose twice daily, morning and evening, throughout the month. You can use this for twenty-five days on and five days off, or you may use it continuously, straight through the month. If your symptoms allow, we recommend taking the five days off because this method more closely mimics your body's own wisdom.

Testosterone: *2.5 to 5.0 milligrams daily,* orally or in a transdermal cream. Use the lowest possible dose.

Optional:

DHEA: 5 to 50 milligrams 1 or 2 times daily, orally or in a transdermal cream, divided doses, twice a day.

All of these hormones can be taken separately or can be compounded into a single product for ease and convenience. We suggest that when combining many products together that you only order a few months' supply at a time to allow for a change in your prescription in the event you and your physician want to modify it.

A recent book, *Hormone of Desire,* by Susan Rako, M.D., a psychiatrist who recommends testosterone replacement for midlife women, which in large measure supports the use of "the naturals," makes the case that when it comes to testosterone, women should make an exception to using "the naturals" and should use the synthetic version, *methyl* testosterone. The author's claim is that since natural testosterone converts to estrogen in the body, while the synthetic doesn't, it is *safer* to use the synthetic. This is not our position. Methyltestosterone is potentially damaging to the liver. The plant-derived bio-identical testosterone is safer on all fronts. In Dr. Laux's experience, even though testosterone can convert to estrogen in some women's bodies, it doesn't seem to do it indiscriminately but rather as a consequence of fulfilling the body's needs and as a result of the body's greater wisdom—part of the beauty of using bio-identicals. If you take testosterone, the simplest way to ensure proper levels is to follow our plan and test your steroid levels, adjusting according to recommended normal parameters, which, for most women, is by reducing the dosage amount and frequency over time as their levels and symptoms stabilize.

Menopause

Joel Hargrove, M.D., chief of the Vanderbilt Menopause Center in Nashville, Tennessee, uses the following medical criteria to determine whether a woman is menopausal:

- estradiol levels are less than 50 picograms/milliliter;
- FSH levels are greater than 50mlU/milligrams; or
- you have no periods for one full year.

For those women who have had the good fortune to reach their mid- to late forties without surgery, there are a number of effective and reliable natural options available, depending on their individual needs and the severity of their symptoms. Again, the type and number of symptoms, as well as their strength and duration, can vary. Some women have symptoms for only a short space of time, while others struggle with menopausal symptoms for many years.

Unlike Provera, a woman using natural progesterone may experience some temporary spotting, which in almost all cases clears up within a few months.

BASIC PROTOCOL

Remifemin, MENO-FEM, or Vitanica Women's Phase II: As directed on the package or by your doctor.

and/or

Progesterone: Alone, *25 to 100 milligrams*—orally or equivalent dose in a transdermal cream, in divided doses twice a day.

If using Pro-Gest® the dose would be

days 1 to 7—do not use cream
days 8 to 21—¼ teaspoon morning and night
days 22 to 31—½ teaspoon morning and night

As symptoms subside, you can gradually begin cutting back on the amount of cream used.

If the above recommendations are not sufficient, or estrogen is needed, we suggest:

Tri-est and progesterone: *1.5 to 5 milligrams total estrogen and 25 to 100 milligrams progesterone* morning and night.

We believe that the tri-est combination will work for most women, but for women who need to use the strongest estrogen, at least temporarily:

Estradiol (E2) and progesterone: *0.5 milligram estradiol, 25 to 100 milligrams progesterone.* After six months try switching to a tri-est formula to lower the estrogen-stimulating effect of taking just E2 and get the protective effects of estriol E3.

Women at High Risk for Cancer, and Breast Cancer Survivors

Here is where the use of estriol and progesterone can be of great benefit to American women. Many of these women are told that they must forego any hormone replacement given the evidence that unopposed estradiol and estrone can increase the risk of breast cancer. But progesterone and estriol have been shown to be potentially *protective* against breast cancer. We recommend that women with a history of cancer, or those who are at high risk for it, use progesterone as part of their hormone therapy even if they are using estriol alone, and regardless of the form of estrogen they are using. Even though estriol has been shown to be protective against cancer and constructively stimulating to the cervix and vaginal tissue, it is nonproliferative in the uterus and breast. And the addition of balancing levels of progesterone is a practice we think prudent until more research is available.

Hopefully, in the future, more doctors will become aware of this protocol. By monitoring serum or saliva progesterone levels and urinary estriol levels, a doctor could determine whether a woman would benefit from this regimen.

BASIC PROTOCOL

Estriol and progesterone: *2 to 5 milligrams* (equivalent in strength to 0.6 to 1.25 milligrams of Premarin) and *25 to 100 milligrams* of progesterone, 2 times a day, morning and evening.

Post-Menopause

It frequently happens that women can pass through their menopause without event and without hormonal imbalance symptoms, but at some time in their sixties they get an osteoporosis test that shows significant bone loss. At this point, estrogen will be prescribed by a doctor in the form of Premarin/Provera because the woman needs "estrogen for her bones." However, in addition to the increased risk of cancer and other side effects, this type of prescription commonly brings on the return of menstruation. Many of these women understandably get quite upset over the fact that they have started bleeding again every month in their sixties. In addition, this course of treatment is not the most effective. Many of these women can do very well on progesterone, diet, exercise, and supplements.

Since both estrogen and progesterone may be needed, a test to determine hormone levels, followed by regular monitoring, is recommended.

BASIC PROTOCOL

Remifemin, MENO-FEM, or Vitanica Women's Phase II: As directed on the package or by your doctor.

and/or:

Progesterone: *25 to 200 milligrams,* in divided doses, morning and evening.

or:

Tri-est and progesterone: *1.5 to 2.5 milligrams total estrogen and 25 to 100 milligrams progesterone* twice a day, morning and evening. Any spotting on this regime will be temporary (no more than a few months).

Topical Preparations

Although the basic principle of the Natural Woman plan is not to treat individual symptoms, there are a number of topical creams that can be used in conjunction with the protocols to more quickly control vaginal dryness or vaginal atrophy. You might want to supplement the program with the following, which can be prepared for you by a compounding pharmacist:

Estriol gel or cream
Estriol cream with added progesterone and testosterone
Vitamin E oil

Staying on the Natural Woman Plan

It is a good idea to get a physical once a year because as your body changes, you will want to keep track of your hormone levels and your osteoporosis risk factors and adjust your prescription accordingly. We have not recommended the use of other hormones, such as DHEA, except for women with surgical menopause, but there is growing interest and research into the value of replenishing this hormone and some women may be interested in consulting their doctor or pharmacist about it.

But, more than anything, when it comes to staying young and vital at midlife, nothing can match paying attention to your diet.

11

HORMONE BALANCING THROUGH FOOD

Fifteen years ago, most conventional doctors would have laughed you out of the office if you told them that broccoli or bran had cancer-preventive properties. Now this is an accepted scientific principle. In fact, a low-fat diet is now an officially sanctioned therapeutic regime for heart disease. Dean Ornish, M.D., one of its primary advocates, had a formidable time at first in making his case. Reversing cardiovascular disease by any means was then considered impossible by the medical profession, and surgery and drugs were the regime of choice. In Dr. Ornish's program, diet, meditation, and yoga, along with social support, are used to reverse heart disease. But you can be sure that convincing conventional medical practitioners that something so ridiculously simple as changing your lifestyle could not only prevent heart disease but could reverse its course was extremely difficult. But with persistence and good science, Dr. Ornish proved the supposedly impossible, and what was quackery then is now considered mainstream medicine.

Today we are just at the beginning of a revolution in how diet is used for the prevention of disease. But most M.D.'s in practice today still don't or can't apply the idea of food as medicine. A survey of doctors done at the Harvard medical school revealed that 90 percent of the doctors surveyed learned their prescription habits from the pharmaceutical salesmen who call on them. These salesmen leave literature and hundreds of samples. Typically, doctors pass the samples along to their patients, and if the patients come back with a positive experience, the doctors will begin writing prescriptions for the drugs for their other patients.

Food as "Medicine" at Midlife

In the same way that "food as medicine" has been (and is still) essentially left out of the protocols for disease prevention in conventional U.S. medical treatment, so has it been in treatment protocols devised for menopausal women. The menopause literature is dominated by the HRT controversy, but little attention is paid to diet. The doctors handing out "little red pills like M&Ms," as described in *Time* magazine, are not advising women on how to use dietary changes to mitigate their symptoms. But, in fact, *diet* may ultimately be the most important factor.

Don't wait around for change to finally get to your doctor's office. In the next ten years there will be an explosion of information as the interest in herbal medicine returns to the front burners of scientific investigation. The National Cancer Institute is already actively promoting a plant-based diet as protection against sex-hormone related cancers (as well as other cancers). But you can get ahead of the curve. You deserve to know right now the latest findings on the benefits of the food you eat on your optimal hormonal health.

In an ideal situation, a woman would not need to take special products to replenish her hormones. If she were eating a plant-based, balanced diet from birth, if the environment didn't tax her body, if she hadn't been hysterectomized, if she weren't on other nutrient-depleting drugs, if, if, if . . . What can't be determined absolutely is that had you been on the Natural Woman eating plan since childhood, would you have avoided hot flashes and night sweats at midlife? Obviously, there will never be a way to know this for certain—but there is clear evidence that points in that direction.

Researchers in Melbourne, Australia, reported in the *British Medical Journal* (October 20, 1990) the results of a study in which they supplemented the normal diets of twenty-five post-menopausal women with phytoestrogen-rich food. After six weeks, those women eating soy flour and linseed (flaxseed) showed signs of a modest estrogen response, accurately assessed by the microscopic examination of vaginal cells. In this case, the phytoestrogen-rich food provided just 10 percent of the women's diets. In Asia, it can be as high as 50 percent, contributing to a minimum of menopausal symptoms and a significant decrease in the incidence of osteoporosis and heart disease.

Plants and Hormonal Health

Again, almost everything we know about hormonal health points back to the wonderful *plant*—to the evolutionary interlinkage between optimum human hormone functioning and the ingesting of a plant-based diet.

Over three hundred known plants possess compounds that have estrogenic activity.[1] Legumes, grains, nuts, and seeds are a rich source of phytoestrogens. There are many different types of phytoestrogens that are structurally similar to human estrogen.

Phytoestrogens either mimic estrogenic activity or affect estrogen metabolism, like the *isoflavones* in soy. Other plant compounds—such as *lignans* found in flaxseed—are not phytoestrogens, but, when ingested, are converted to biologically active estrogenic substances. Your intestinal bacteria can change some food compounds, such as the lignans in flaxseed, into hormonally active substances that your body can then use. These plant compounds work in your body by raising or lowering your hormone levels as needed. You might say that they naturally help control your hormonal rheostat. And other substances in these plant foods offer the additional benefits of immune fortification, including protection from cancer and support of the body's elimination of toxins.

In addition, there are hundreds of other chemicals naturally occurring in plant foods that are variously and interchangeably known as *phytochemicals, phytonutrients, or nutraceuticals.* These substances are not classified as vitamins, minerals, fiber, or complex carbohydrates, but they are vital for your good health. To drive the point home: At least 150 studies around the world have shown that people who eat the most fruits and vegetables are half as likely to have cancer as those who eat the least.[2] In over a hundred human studies, the eating of some food from plants is associated with a lower risk of some type of cancer.

Does this mean that you should become a vegetarian? Not necessarily. But there is a great deal of evidence demonstrating that your diet should lean heavily in that direction. It's been shown that vegetarians have lower levels of estradiol and estrone within the normal range, which is related to fewer menopausal symptoms and a lower incidence of cancer. A diet high in animal fat gives you higher estrogen levels, which are associated with a greater incidence of menopausal complications, cancers, and all the other degenerative diseases. High animal-food intake and low plant-food intake create an internal imbalance that is associated with an increase in menopausal problems and disease in general. A plant-rich diet appears to have a hormone-regulating effect and can be protective against xenoestrogens, while an animal-rich diet is associated with increased danger from elevated estrogen, among other undesirable and health-compromising factors.

Just by our lunch and dinner choices we affect our hormonal health. The food you eat is a *control system* for all your hormonal systems—not for just the sex hormones. You must remember that everything you are starts from *food, air,* and *water.* You eat it, you digest it, you absorb it, and that becomes your blood. Your blood nourishes your glands, and your glands pull in the nutrients they need in order to make hormones. The food you eat can create hormonal health or hormonal havoc.

Your Genes Have Less Influence Than Your Diet

A great deal of medical research has been done on how much your genes can affect your risk of getting various forms of cancer. Now scientists are discovering that diet is at least as important, if not more so.

Cancer rates and types vary worldwide geographically. In China, cancer is not widespread. In fact, it occurs in specific areas as a local disease, and its incidence ranges from very high to practically none.

The villagers have relatively uniform genetic backgrounds because they remain in the location of their birth. But diet can differ greatly from village to village. And, indeed, it's in these dietary differences that researchers are finding valuable clues. Hereditary factors are far less implicated in causing cancer than previously thought, and diet is more important than most suspected.

The Oxford-Cornell China Diet and Health Project

This study, headed by T. Colin Campbell of Cornell University, is the largest, most comprehensive study ever done to determine precisely how diet and lifestyle affect disease. In 6,500 people across China, 367 dietary, health, and lifestyle factors were evaluated. This study stands out singularly in its importance because it assessed the effects of different foods and lifestyle habits on a genetically homogeneous population. Outside the major cities in China, 90 percent of the population doesn't leave the region they were born in, and each region has its own local produce, dietary preferences, and personal habits. These diets and customs vary enormously from region to region, revealing different disease prevalences. What this study showed was the health benefits or detriments of a variety of specific lifestyle choices.

First and foremost, the study definitively showed the great benefit of a predominantly plant-based diet, which is nutrient-rich, high in fiber, and low in fat content. Most Americans eat a diet that contains only 30 percent vegetables and fruit, whereas the study details the benefits of an 80 to 100 percent plant-based diet. In general, vegetarians have 40 percent less risk of cancer, 30 percent less risk of heart disease from reduced blood flow, and 20 percent less risk of mortality overall.

The study clearly demonstrated the *protective* value of eating a diet rich in a variety of plant foods, in as close to their natural state as possible. The people in the study who ate the highest amount of plant foods were the healthiest and had the lowest incidence of cancer. This diet was protective of a number of sex hormone–related cancers, including, among others, breast and prostate cancer. The study also showed us that *less fat in the diet overall* is very important for lowering cholesterol and protecting against heart disease, since excess fat in the diet seems to interfere with the way in which hormones interact with each other.

To prevent cancer and many other degenerative diseases, less is best when it comes to animal products—and a lot less is even better. First, saturated fat from animal products can lead to high cholesterol levels and is associated with increased cancer incidence. The China project found that the higher the serum cholesterol levels, the higher the number of deaths from stomach, esophageal, lung, colon and rectal cancers, and leukemia. For example, women in an area with the highest serum cholesterol levels showed a 473 percent increase in deaths from esophageal cancer alone. Men showed similar increases.

There are other suspected links between diet and certain cancers, as early results of the study show a relationship between animal fat and breast cancer. And it appears that the lower your cholesterol, the lower your risk of getting not only cancer, but many other diseases as well. The Chinese have far lower cholesterol levels than we do. The high end of their cholesterol range is our lowest: Compare a range of 88 to 165 in China against 160 to 340 or more in the United States. Fat makes up only 15 percent of the average person's daily dietary calories in China. That is two thirds less fat than we eat.

In addition, the China project showed that animal protein is also related to higher cancer rates. People who eat a lot of animal protein have greater amounts of bile salts in their colon. These higher levels are thought to contribute to colo-rectal cancer. Women with high serum protein levels showed higher death rates from stomach and esophageal cancers. There was also more leukemia and lung cancer among people who ate lots of animal protein.

The Chinese consume one third less protein than we do overall. In fact, in many areas, all their protein is of plant origin. But, westernization of their diet is spreading out from the cities. Now, for instance, in certain regions 93 percent of their protein intake is from plants and 7 percent from animals. The data from the China project shows that just this seemingly minor 7 percent increase in animal protein intake was enough to cause an increase in the cancer incidence in those regions. Americans eat ten times more animal protein than that.

The average daily intake of fiber for participants in the China project was thirty-four grams. Ours is around ten grams of fiber per day. After lung cancer, colorectal cancers claim the most lives of people who die from cancer. Fiber may be very protective here. Adding fiber to your diet has been shown in other studies to actually shrink precancerous polyps in the lower colon, thus reducing your cancer risk.

Fiber is known to help keep your elimination regular and to support a healthy intestinal environment. In women, a lack of fiber in the diet can cause the estrogen that is destined to be excreted to be reabsorbed and reused, potentially putting you at risk for estrogen dominance.[3]

The Advantages of an Asian Diet

Based on the results of the Oxford-Cornell China Diet and Health Project, and other examinations of the Asian diet and aboriginal diets, there is ample reason to believe that a good proportion of symptomatic women (excluding those whose hormones were surgically intervened with) may be so because of past dietary practices and nutritional deficit, and would do well to look at the traditional diets of Asian countries. One ingredient in the Asian diet that seems key is soy. The average Japanese consumes fifty to eighty grams (two to three ounces) of soy per day. The average American consumes five grams of soy a day—mostly obtained in poor forms, such as in the additives in margarines and salad dressings, which contain harmful fats and preservatives as well as other undesirable ingredients.

The Special Power of Soy

Soy is a food that has powerful, proven, anticancer and longevity properties and is the new darling of the nutritional community. In scientific language, soy contains genistein, daidzein, protease inhibitor, phytate, saponins, phytosterols, phenolic acids, and lecithin, as well as other still to be discovered compounds. It has been shown to be an inhibitor of breast and prostate cancer, and it is now being studied extensively for a potential new type of anticancer drug. Soy has also been identified as the prime factor in why Asian women with a diet heavily reliant on it don't experience menopausal symptoms.

From the mainstream journal *Primary Care & Cancer* comes this information:

> Researchers looking into the disease prevention qualities of plant foods like soybeans and green tea credit compounds that may work like estrogen as one reason for the benefits. Research has shown that the most potent of these compounds have about 0.5% of the activity of your natural estrogens. Of these phytoestrogens, the two categories creating the most furor are isoflavonoids and flavonoids—especially an isoflavonoid known as *genistein.* . . . Epidemiological evidence indicates that Asian women have a lower incidence of breast and colon cancer, better response to cancer treatment, and fewer problems with menopause than Western women. And among the apparent reasons for this is that Asians, in general, consume more soy products—tofu included—and green tea . . . "I guess I'm going to have to learn to eat soybean meal and drink tea . . . and become an Oriental woman . . ." says Cyrus R. Creeling of the National Institute of Diabetes and Digestive and Kidney Diseases on the powerful benefits of the Asian diet.[4]

Moreover, British scientists recently announced that the *isoflavonoids* in soy may help prevent breast cancer, and that ways are being developed to enhance soy proteins to increase their anticancer properties.[5]

Tofu, made from soy, may beat out spinach as the food Americans most want to say "yuck!" to, but this plant-derived food has been proven to be exceptionally beneficial to health. True, it's certainly easier to take an HRT pill than give up the daily burger and fries and coffee on the run. But what you put in your mouth has a greater impact on your health than anyone ever anticipated. For example, by just adding soy to your diet, your levels of LH and FSH hormones would show a beneficial modification—and that's just one food!

Will some women who've lived on less than perfect diets for most of their lives get through menopause without symptoms or live to a ripe old age free of disease? Of course. Every constitution is different, but statistically and practically you'll find yourself on the wrong side of the tracks when you don't follow a plant-based diet. And no one should forego the positive, protective powers of plants when it comes to disease prevention. Following a plant-rich diet is easier than you think, and there are many ways to create inviting and flavorful meals for yourself and your family.

Not Just a "Lady's" Diet

This diet is healthy for everyone. Your spouse/boyfriend/male friend/son/grandson can join you in this basic diet, as the balancing effects of plant foods on hormones in men is good for all sorts of modern maladies, including sex hormone–related diseases such as prostate cancer. A recent study found that *isoflavones* from soy and other plants are *tyrosine kinase inhibitors* for specific tissues such as the prostate cell. Tyrosine kinase enzymes are secreted by malignant cells. This may further explain some of the correlation between soy ingestion and a lower incidence of breast cancer and prostate cancer when eating the traditional Asian diet.[6] In the United States, the incidence of prostate cancer in men is the same as the incidence of breast cancer in women, suggesting to researchers that these diseases share a common mechanism in tissues that are of the same embryological origin but are differentiated by gender.[7]

Herman Aldercreutz, M.D., one of the foremost investigators in this area, did studies relating to the incidence of prostate cancer in Japanese men. Japanese men who had high phytosterol levels in their blood did not get prostate cancer.[8] Protect all the men in your life by getting them to join you on a plant-rich diet.

Good Digestion Is Crucial to Hormonal Health

You can be eating all the right things for your hormonal health, but if you're not digesting properly, you won't be maximizing your benefits. If your intestinal health is poor, then your overall health is compromised, according to clinical and historical observations and the latest scientific data.

Good digestion starts with chewing your food well for an efficient and thorough food breakdown in your stomach and small intestine, where most nutrients are absorbed. If you experience gas, constipation, diarrhea, bloating, can't eat much at one time, food seems to sit in your stomach too long, you have a poorly formed stool, or you have any other digestive complaints, you need to improve your digestive vigor. Ironically, women who take a lot of antacids to combat their symptoms of poor digestion are actually interfering with their ability to convert phytoestrogens and lignans from plants and make them more hormonally viable.

We recommend plant digestive enzymes (see chapter 13 for further information) for any woman who wants to enhance her digestion. Taking two to three plant digestive enzyme capsules at the beginning of your meals will help your system to fully break down, digest, and absorb the valuable nutrients in your food. They will aid in easing your digestive challenges and will improve your functioning.

Here is a fundamental idea that is rarely brought up for the midlife woman: The relative health of your intestines determines whether you make beneficial active substances from your food or whether you make toxins. The health and balance of your intestinal flora is very important. We naturally have many hundreds of different species of intestinal microbes that live in harmony in our intestines. We absolutely need them for our health as they are responsible for such important tasks as helping make antibodies, utilizing certain vitamins, and even rendering carcinogens harmless. In order to maintain a healthy population of these organisms, we need to do what a farmer does—nourish the "soil" of our intestines.

If we have poor intestinal health, we can cause an imbalance of our intestinal inhabitants, and pathogenic bacteria can proliferate and then compromise our health. One way they can do this is by converting estrogens destined for elimination into a reabsorbable form, at which point they can put you at higher risk for estrogen-sensitive cancers.

In our chapter on supplements (chapter 13), we will direct you toward finding insightful tests that can determine your specific digestive needs, and we will suggest supplements to improve and balance your digestion.

Never Too Late

From the youngest woman reading this book to the oldest: Start now. It is never too early or too late to start eating right. A young woman on a healthy plant-based diet may never experience any of the frustrating symptoms of her older sisters, and may be one of those lucky ones whose cessation of menstruation is but a blip on the screen. For older women, they will be doing much to ensure a healthy, vigorous, sexy, and disease-free old age.

12

THE NATURAL WOMAN EATING PLAN

Does anyone expect you to be perfect? To follow this eating plan to the letter? Of course not.

But if you adhered to it by only 10 percent, if you began to take some of the principles and added them into your regular habits, you would be making an important change in your hormonal health.

And remember: A diet good for menopause is also good for your overall health.

If your overall eating pattern changes . . . If you begin principally to add in the greens, the phytosterol-rich vegetables, and to get rid of the Fritos and the diet sodas . . . If you have added in exercise . . . You've then gone a long way toward both improving your overall health and mollifying the menopause passage. And if you got up to 50 percent, you might find that the benefits were so great, your whole approach to eating would have changed. You would begin to see that what you take into your body is reflected in how you feel and what you see in the mirror. Does this mean you can never have a cup of coffee, or a piece of delicious apple tart, or a glass of red wine? Not at all. Just change your approach and see these foods as treats. Moderate your usage.

How to Eat for Hormonal Health

Here are the fundamental principles to follow to add to your daily diet. (In appendixes E and F, we will list recommended brands and resources for organic products and a number of excellent cookbooks that will help you adapt these principles to recipes.)

A BASICALLY PLANT-BASED DIET

This is the centerpiece of the Natural Woman plan: that is, vegetables, grains, legumes, fruits, seeds, nuts, and sea vegetables. Americans tend to average only two and a half servings of these daily—half the recommended daily allowance. At about half a cup per serving, we are eating only about one and a half servings of vegetables, less than one serving of fruit, and less than a third of a serving of legumes or nuts. So start by stepping up the quantity and variety of your consumption of fruits and vegetables in your daily diet.

The fiber in the plants you eat is just as important as the nutrients. In a woman's diet, a lack of fiber in the diet can cause estrogen to be reabsorbed and recycled.

FRESH, WHOLE, UNREFINED, AND UNPROCESSED FOODS

Get the absolute most out of your food: Choose certified organic produce whenever possible. Organic farming, which is the growing and producing of natural foods without the use of synthetic fertilizers, pesticides, or chemical additives, is the fastest growing segment in commercial agriculture today. Our increasing awareness of the dangers of toxic chemicals has created an unprecedented demand for safe and more nourishing organic foods. Organically grown fruits and vegetables are grown in more nutrient-rich soils, taste better, and are without the chemical baggage of their commercial counterparts. Supermarkets that carry organic foods are now sprouting up in mainstream American life. You will find that the produce tastes better and that the cost is quite affordable. Prices have come down markedly in the last few years. Even mainstream markets are now upgrading and include more natural foods, free of pesticides and synthetic additives.

TRY TO EAT SEASONAL AND REGIONAL AS MUCH AS POSSIBLE

Besides the value of providing the potentially freshest and best-tasting produce available, eating seasonal and regional has many health benefits. All animals eat their food in their own region, and eat what each season offers. A region is affected by its specific seasonal climate and soil condition, and eating fresh food in a natural rotation and in variety has nutritional and phytochemical protections. Traditional cultures eating seasonal and regional diets suffer less from the chronic health problems or menopausal distresses than do modern cultures that have the "advantages" of refrigeration and the ability to eat foods out of season shipped from other regions around the world.

WHOLE GRAIN FOODS

Stick with whole grains whenever possible. They have higher fiber and phytosterol content, which is not true of refined foods, and they are major sources of minerals like magnesium, zinc, and chromium. Refined flours are poor in nutrients and readily metabolize into sugars. Whole grains offer greater nutrition for providing sustained energy and can taste a world apart.

NO ADDITIVES, COLORINGS, OR PRESERVATIVES

This is extremely important. These substances can be allergenic and toxic and many are carcinogenic. You want to eat *clean, safe, whole, and wholesome* food. In this way you can avoid possible environmental contamination as well as intentionally manufactured technological nonfood substances. One of the toxins this will help you avoid is xenoestrogens—chemicals such as pesticides and plastics that can actually have estrogenic activity in your body and can alter your hormonal balance.

EAT A VARIETY OF FOODS

No one food or nutrient can do it all for you. You want to get the protective benefit of phytochemicals from a wide range of foods, taking advantage of each plant's *unique* nutritional and phytochemical attributes and biological strategies. The cumulative synergistic effect of "the team" is far superior to any single megadosing of a food or nutrient.

EAT MEAT SPARINGLY

Meat has too much saturated fat, is low in nutrients, has few antioxidants and no fiber, and is calorie dense. Too much fat in the diet can increase your risk of any number of cancers and heart disease, so stick with fish, poultry, and wild game and eat red meat (including pork) infrequently.

Begin to reduce your consumption of meat by eating smaller portions, as if the meat were a condiment to your vegetables, pastas, and grains. Increase your consumption of fish, particularly cold-water fish such as salmon, tuna, halibut, and mackerel. These fish contain the valuable omega-3 essential fatty acids, which your body doesn't make for itself. Essential fatty acids are involved in hormone production as well as in protecting your heart and arteries from oxidative damage. The best concentrated vegetable source of EFAs is flaxseed.

ELIMINATE JUNK FOOD

We're not asking you to give up potato or tortilla chips, but we are recommending that you buy better quality products that are available in natural food markets and in the natural foods sections of many major chains. Almost any comfort food or favorite snack you love and can't live without has a safer, healthier version now available. These natural versions are made with real food ingredients, while the commercial brands are often a conglomerate of refined and synthetic chemicals and unnecessary additives, with no nutritional or health benefit, and worse still, potential health threats. The natural products are low in fat, they're baked, not fried, and they're made without hydrogenated oils and preservatives. If you haven't been paying attention and think "health food" substitutes aren't as good as the standard brands, take another look, because there are now many excellent choices available, and many of the natural products are *better* tasting.

EXERCISE CAUTION WITH MILK PRODUCTS

Beyond the fact that some people are lactose intolerant and that milk is no longer considered the "perfect food" that supplies all the necessary nutrients for a good diet,[1] there are many reasons to avoid commercial milk products. Farmers use numerous antibiotics in dairy farming, plus pesticides in the field, and the residue of these products has been found in milk, leading to potential health threats such as exposing you to antibiotic-resistant bacteria. In addition, in 1993, the government approved the use of rBGH (recombinant bovine growth hormone) to increase production despite many doubts among health professionals about its safety for humans. If you are not lactose intolerant, choose organic milk, the low-fat or skim variety. There are now a number of organic milk producers around the country, and the number is growing. The price is slightly higher, but it is definitely worth the extra cost. If you eat cheese, eat real cheese and only occasionally, as the fat content is very high. Use real organic cultured low-fat yogurt. For greater health benefits, substitute soy or rice milk beverages as often as possible. Those of you brought up on milk might be initially resistant to these other "milks," but there are a number of good-tasting brands on the market. To start, try substituting them in cereal. They can also be used in sauces where milk or cream is called for (see appendix E for recommended brands).

AVOID FRIED FOODS

Steam, broil, bake, poach, boil, sauté in light oil, and quick stir-fry whenever possible. Try to keep your daily calories from fat at 15 percent. Avoid using saturated fats like lard, shortenings, and partially hydrogenated oils like margarine. They contain unnaturally created *trans-fatty acids,* which are carcinogenic and pose many other serious health hazards. When using butter, try the organic kind, or we recommend a clarified butter called *ghee* that can be purchased in health food stores. As already noted, a high-fat diet has a negative impact on your hormonal metabolism.

USE SEED-BASED OILS

Look for organic oils such as olive, canola, sesame, safflower, hazelnut, and walnut. Organic oils are free of the harmful chemicals used in processing. In the case of olive oil, buy extra-virgin, which is unrefined and therefore has more nutrients. These fresh organic oils should smell like the nut or seed from which they are pressed. Traditionally, oils were pressed fresh and delivered on a weekly basis; they didn't sit on shelves for years at a time. Our recommendation is to buy organic oils fresh, refrigerate them, then use them in moderation and replace them regularly.

FOODS BEST KEPT TO A MINIMUM

Certain foods are known to aggravate hormonal imbalance symptoms, and, in excess, can compromise your overall health.

Caffeine. Drinking coffee leeches calcium from your bones and can be very stressful to your system. Many women experience increased frequency and intensity of hot flashes when they drink coffee. Although it has some caffeine, choose green tea instead. Green tea has a mildly stimulating effect without giving you the jitters, and provides potent phytochemical and antioxidant protections. Black tea is also preferable, as it has phytosterol benefits. Also, choose herbal teas whenever possible. If you do drink coffee, try organic coffee, which is less acidic and has a superior taste.

Refined sugar. Sugars are not inherently bad. We need them to live, which should be welcome news to women who think they can't live without them. But *refined* sugars contain empty calories and create an acidic internal environment, which, like coffee, leeches minerals from your bones. The refining of any food removes valuable nutrients and turns a health-promoting food into a disease-promoting food.

Women at high risk for osteoporosis should particularly avoid foods with refined sugar. There is also evidence that the disregulation of a woman's blood sugar levels from eating too much refined sugar can contribute to hot flashes.

But there are many healthy ways to *sweeten* your life. We recommend raw honey (real and organic), real maple syrup, brown rice syrup, organic molasses, or Sucanat. Sucanat (natural sugarcane) is a whole sugarcane product that is totally unrefined and only minimally processed, meaning that the nutrients are left in and the food value remains. It is an excellent substitute for refined sugar in your drinks and in baking.

Table salt. Like sugar, you don't need to completely eliminate salt from your diet to eat healthily, but table salt is highly refined and contains unhealthy anti-caking agents, sugars, and flowing agents. Even most sea salts sold in health food stores have been refined and do not have their original healthful benefits. We recommend the product Celtic Sea Salt, which not only tastes great as a condiment and in your cooking, but also contains eighty-four minerals and trace elements. Its mineral content and balance are very similar to your own blood's mineral salt composition.

Alcohol. Despite the numerous health benefits cited for moderate alcohol consumption, particularly red wine, women at midlife should stay on the low-moderate side of alcohol consumption, as alcohol can aggravate hormonal imbalance symptoms. Women who have more than two drinks a day increase their risk of osteoporosis. Hard liquor should be avoided altogether. Try to limit yourself to a glass of wine or beer on occasion (organic products are available). Red wine is preferable to white, as studies have shown that the phytosterol components of grape skin, which is removed for white wine, help to lower cholesterol, raise HDL ("good" cholesterol) levels, and reduce the risk of heart disease. Actually, further studies have shown that you can get similar health benefits from just drinking unfermented grape (not white) juice.

Diet sodas and soft drinks. When it comes to your bones (and, for that matter, your overall health), diet sodas and soft drinks have a high phosphorus content, which is a real threat to their integrity. High phosphorus intake creates internal imbalance and causes minerals to be leeched from your bones. The synthetic sweeteners in diet sodas and in other products should be avoided as well, as they pose their own health risks.

Chocolate and cocoa. These are wonderful comfort foods that need to be limited to the status of a treat. Because they contain refined sugars (and fats and additives), these foods have been known to increase hot flashes. There are excellent organic chocolates and cocoas available made with real ingredients, not synthetic additives, and sweetened with Sucanat (see appendix E).

Excessively spicy foods. For some women, Indian and Mexican cuisine can induce hot flashes, so be advised. But, on the whole, these are fine and are recommended cuisines as long as you watch the fats and lards.

Cigarettes. Smoking cigarettes is the number-one preventable cause of cancer and the leading preventable cause of overall mortality and morbidity. Avoid absolutely, for every health reason we can think of. Among its many negatives, smoking lowers native estrogen levels. An interesting caveat is that the Japanese have a very high per capita smoking rate but also have a much lower than expected cancer rate. The reason? It is theorized that the protective effect of their plant-based diet, including their soy foods and green tea, is responsible.

Plant Foods with Known Phytosterol Activity[2]

Eating a variety of vegetables, legumes, herbs, and spices can give you significant dietary support for easing menopausal discomfort. These plant foods have many other positive attributes in addition to their phytosterol content—including antioxidant and phytochemical protection—that enhance your health and immunity.

The study of phytosterols in food is a growing scientific field and new information about their multiple benefits for the human diet appears daily. Some plants are considered "estrogenic," and stimulate your estrogen receptors. Others are considered progesterogenic, and stimulate your progesterone receptors. Phytosterols can help you self-regulate; that is, they will "up" your estrogen or progesterone if needed, or lower it if needed. The idea here is that these dietary factors can help balance and support your hormonal well-being gently, naturally, and effectively.

Here is a list of foods with known phytosterol activity to incorporate in your daily diet:

VEGETABLES

artichoke, Jerusalem
asparagus
bamboo shoot
beans (common, seedlings, kidney with pods, immature mung, sprouts)
beet
brussel sprout
cabbage

carrot
cauliflower
celery
chive
corn
cucumber
eggplant
garlic
green beans
lettuce
mustard greens
okra
onion
parsley
pea seedling
pepper (red, green, yellow, orange)
potato (all kinds)
pumpkin
radish
seaweed
shallot
soybean
spinach
taro
tomato
turnip
yam

FRUITS
apple
apricot
banana
cherry
date
fig
grape
grapefruit
lemon
muskmelon

orange
peach
pear
pineapple
plum
pomegranate
strawberry
watermelon

CEREALS AND GRAINS

barley
buckwheat
corn
millet
rice
rice bran
rye
sorghum
wheat (bran, flour, whole)

LEGUMES (BEANS)

azuki
broad
chickpea
kidney
mung
sasage
pea
peanut
soybean

SEEDS AND NUTS

almond
cashew
coconut
pecan
pine nut
pistachio
sesame seed

sunflower seed
walnut

MOST COMMON OILS

coconut
corn
linseed (flaxseed)
olive
peanut
rice bran
safflower
sesame seed
soybean
sunflower
walnut
wheat germ

EGGS

In the scheme of the food chain, a fresh, organic egg provides powerful nutrition and has phytosterol content. The yolk contains many potent enzymes and is rich in DNA. But yolks are high in fats and can hold concentrates of pesticides and environmental contaminants, which is why it is important to stick with organic products and to limit consumption. But the total food value of the egg is undeniable.

BEER

The hops in beer have a high phytosterol content. Beer is made from grains, malts, herbs, active yeast, and water. Any time a food is fermented, its absorbability is enhanced, improving its nutritional qualities. In Europe, dark beers known to be rich in nutrients have been used for centuries to enrich a woman's breast milk and to improve her health and stamina. Along with red wine, beer has been shown to have health-protective qualities and can be consumed in moderation.

ADD MORE SPICE TO YOUR LIFE

Unfortunately, American cooking tends to be very short on these wonderful condiments, but spices have known phytosterol activity and can help balance your hormones. Garlic, in particular, has multiple benefits for your health. It is interesting to note that the country with the lowest incidence of cancer is India, and this has been attributed to the fact that the people in India use a great *number* and a great *variety* of spices in their diets. Dr. David Heber of the National Cancer Institute urges all Americans to literally add more spice for a more healthful life. We agree. Use herbs and spices fresh, whenever possible or suitable, as a bottle of spice that has been sitting in your spice rack for fifteen years is unlikely to have much benefit. And the more variety of spices the better. Variety brings out the virtues of many different plants working together for your body. Commonly used spices with phytosterol activity are:

allspice
caraway
cardamom
cinnamon
clove
coriander
cumin
dill
fennel
garlic
ginger
licorice
mace
marjoram
nutmeg
oregano
paprika
pepper
rosemary
sage
savory
tarragon
thyme
turmeric

SEA VEGETABLES

Here the Asians have benefited greatly in their health because of their use of plant foods from the sea. In an Asian diet, seaweeds are very common ingredients in main dishes or are mixed with vegetables or rice dishes, soups, and salads.

There are literally hundreds of varieties of sea vegetables, or seaweed, which contain all the known essential minerals and trace elements needed for proper nutrition. They are an excellent source of vegetable protein and are very low in fat. Sea vegetables are all usually less than 2 percent fat, and the fat they do have is the protective, healthy kind, the omega-3s.

For Westerners, sea vegetables usually take some getting used to. They can look and taste "weird," especially if not prepared properly. But those with a taste for Japanese sushi rolls wrapped in *nori* seaweed have already made a start in the sea vegetable direction, and many of you will find that you can develop a real taste for them.

One of their assets is their high mineral content, without which your body can't regulate your hormones or maintain your nervous system. Each sea vegetable has its own unique properties. *Hijiki,* for example, is particularly high in calcium and iron. One cup of hijiki contains more calcium than half a cup of milk, and more iron than two eggs. A mere one-half ounce of *dulse* will more than satisfy your daily thyroid requirement for iodine. (However, if you avoid iodine-containing foods, then you should avoid sea vegetables.) And sea vegetables can protect you from the ill effects of radon and pollution and help to purify your body of toxins.[3] *Kombu, wakame, arame, hijiki,* and other kelp family members contain a phytochemical called sodium alginate, which can reduce the absorption of radioactive strontium by 50 to 80 percent. Extracts from sea vegetables, principally carrageenan and agar, are an integral part of today's processed foods, and are found in such foods as ice creams, baked goods, salad dressings, and yogurts, but have limited benefit in these forms.

Sea vegetables can be found in health food stores and ethnic markets. Once you gain some familiarity with them, they are very easy to add to your favorite soups, salads, casseroles, and stews.

SUPER SOY—IT'S MORE THAN JUST LEARNING TO LOVE TOFU

This bland white stuff packs a powerful punch when it comes to balancing and replenishing hormones and has demonstrated cancer-preventive properties. Eat some tofu every day. Try to do what the Japanese do and eat at least three ounces a day. Its very blandness makes it easy to take, easy to mask, easy to make. Marinate it with your favorite flavors—herbs or spices—and bake it or grill it. Cut it up and put it in your salads or put it in scrambled eggs and pasta sauces. Use soy milk beverage instead of cow's milk in cereal. Soy milk is very bland, but a soy milk beverage like vanilla soy milk can be delicious and goes great with cereal or with your snacks (see appendix E for recommended brands). You will be amazed at how well it will adapt to your diet. Want a delicious chocolate pudding? Nori-mu makes one from a chocolate soy milk beverage. The same company makes nondairy cream pies. Want a hot chocolate? Heat soy milk with cocoa.

As a condiment, tamari is preferable to soy sauce, as it has a higher phytosterol content. You can make *miso* soup at home, quickly and simply, and add your favorite herbs and vegetables to it. It literally takes minutes to make, and this fermented soybean preparation is as healthy as it is tasty. And try a tempeh burger. Tempeh is a soybean product that is heartier and heavier than tofu, with a more meatlike texture.

CALCIUM-RICH FOODS

There are many ways to get sufficient calcium in your diet without resorting to calcium pills and milk products (see chapter 14). In our chapter on osteoporosis, you will learn about the importance of other minerals, such as magnesium, for the health of your bones. Here is a list of calcium-rich foods. The calcium content is based on 3½-ounce portions, and the amount in milligrams is approximate.

Hijiki*	1,400 milligrams
Wakame*	1,300
Kelp*	1,100
Kombu*	800
Brick cheese	680

Wheat or barley grass	515
Sardines	445
Agar agar*	400
Nori*	260
Sesame seeds (hulled)	200 to 300
Almonds	235
Soybeans (dried)	225
Amaranth	220
Canned salmon (with bones)	200 to 250
Hazelnuts	210
Parsley	200
Turnip greens	190
Collard greens	190
Brazil nuts	185
Dandelion greens	185
Kale	185
Sunflower seeds	175
Watercress	150
Garbanzo beans	150
White beans (dried)	145
Quinoa	140
Mustard greens	140
Black beans	135
Pinto beans (dried)	135
Broccoli	130
Yogurt	120
Milk	120
Beet greens	120
Tofu	115
Chinese cabbage	105
Spinach (cooked)	105
Walnuts	85
Okra	80
Cottage cheese	60
Eggs	55
Brown rice	35
Bluefish	25
Halibut	15
Chicken	10

Ground beef	10
Mackerel	5

*sea vegetables

What to Drink

Drink plenty of water all day long. Try for at least six 8-ounce glasses a day. Also buy natural spring water whenever possible. It is better than distilled water, which contains none of the natural minerals. Avoid unfiltered tap water, as it can be contaminated with chemicals and even viruses and bacteria.

Fruit juices. Fresh are best. Don't overdo them. Most commercial fruit juices are not real fruit and contain too much refined sugar. You can drink them diluted occasionally.

Soy drinks. Many soy beverage drinks are now available in natural food markets. Some are better than others, so don't be discouraged if the first one you try is not great tasting (see appendix E for recommendations).

Rice drinks. As with soy, there is a variety of rice beverage drinks that can be very tasty, such as amazake, flavored (almond, pecan, vanilla, mocha java) cultured rice drinks that can be delicious.

Herbal teas and green teas. These can be drunk iced or hot.

Beer and wine. These can be drunk on occasion. Natural and organic beers and wines are available and are preferred not only for flavor but for health. Avoid hard liquor.

An Everyday Eating Plan

Now, how would the basic principles of the Natural Woman eating plan translate into what you eat every day? Does it sound like a challenge? Change often is, particularly if your diet is all fast food on the run. But you will be amazed at how easily and painlessly this diet can be incorporated into your daily routine.

BEST CHOICES FOR BREAKFAST

Oatmeal, dried cereals (natural, without added sugar), muesli—substitute soy or rice milk beverage for low-fat milk whenever possible
Whole grain bread, plain or toasted, with small amount of butter or nut butter and/or all-fruit jam
Fruit—fresh or dried
Low-fat yogurt
Eggs—limit to six per week
Herbal teas, green tea. Green tea, though it contains some caffeine, has powerful antioxidant factors. Choose it over coffee. But if you do drink coffee, organic coffee is tastier and healthier than regular commercial coffees.

BEST CHOICES FOR LUNCH

Vegetable salads of all kinds
Tuna, salmon, sardines, chicken, turkey
Eggs, tofu, soy cheese
Tomato
Whole grain breads
Fruits
Water
Herbal or green tea
Sparkling fruit drinks
Limit mayonnaise, oils

BEST CHOICES FOR DINNER

Steamed or poached fish, grilled or baked chicken or turkey, pasta, brown rice, wild rice, potatoes
Leafy green vegetables
All vegetables listed above with diced tofu mixed in

BEST CHOICES FOR DESSERT

Many desserts can be adapted to provide more overall nutrition. Use fruit juices in place of sugar. Use whole wheat flour. Adapt custard recipes by using soy products. Many packaged cookies (see appendix E) are made without refined sugar.

Fresh fruits
Frozen yogurt

Frozen fruit sorbets
Honey and Sucanat-sweetened whole grain cookies
Nori-mu pudding
Rice dream, a frozen ice-creamlike dessert. Comes in pints, bars, and sandwiches
Organic chocolate

Staying on the Eating Plan

Remember, don't think you must deprive yourself completely or approach this plan as a *diet* for losing weight. The feeling of deprivation is the first step to falling off the plan. Don't forget to treat yourself on occasion. Fortunately, when you are eating *real* food, it is actually hard to overeat in terms of calories. What you will normally experience is that you feel full and sated long before you could do any calorie damage. When you eat refined foods, you can consume too many calories from fats and sugars very quickly because the nutrition, fiber, and bulk are not present. Follow your intuition and not a calorie chart. Eat well and eat hearty.

13

SUPPLEMENTS: FOR HORMONAL AND OVERALL HEALTH

Adhering to the Natural Woman eating plan and sticking with fresh, organic food as much as possible is the first line of defense, but you are going to give yourself that much more protection against our strenuous environment if you begin to take supplements. Commercially produced foods, which are lacking in essential nutrients and contain unwanted pesticides and chemicals, further complicate our health concerns. This applies to men as well; except for the specific vitamin supplements that provide an emphasis on a woman's particular needs, men can use these same recommendations.

Supplements are intended to do just that: *supplement,* not replace, a healthy diet. But when added to what you eat, they can improve not only your hormonal health but your overall well-being, including your immune system and your level of energy.

Multivitamins and Minerals

The foundation of the Natural Woman supplement plan is a broad-spectrum multivitamin and mineral complex that fills in any nutritional voids. Many vitamins are essential, meaning that they must come from our diets because we don't manufacture them ourselves. In a healthy body, there are some vitamins, like those in the B vitamin family, that we can actually make ourselves. Minerals, however, must come from our diets. The way in which commercial foods are refined and the nutrient-poor soil in which they are grown depletes their mineral content. Without minerals, vitamins can't work. Minerals act like a spark plug because they are used in many enzyme pathways and bring about processes in the body such as digestion and the making of red and white blood cells, to name just two. Without active enzymes, these body functions would not take place no matter how many vitamins you took. Whether minerals are needed in large or minute amounts, they are mandatory in helping to create and protect your health. We include on our list several products that are specifically designed for osteoporosis and a woman's hormonal balance.

In general, we don't recommend single supplements. Nutrientswork together as a team. Taking a high dose of a single nutrient will not, in most cases, make up for a deficiency of another. If a person takes a single nutrient in abundance, instead of correcting an imbalance they can actually create more of an imbalance in the system.

Brands we recommend:

Prevail's Advance Multi Vitamin and Mineral
Naturally's Super Herbalized Vita Boost II
Ethical Nutrients' Multi Nutrients
Enzymatic Therapy's Biovital
Solgar Formula VM 75
Tyler Encapsulations' Multiplex II
PhytoPharmica's Bio-Essential or Clinical Nutrients for women
Rx Vitamins' ReVitalize

Enchanced mineral content for treating osteoporosis:

Prevail's Osteo Formula
Tyler Encapsulations' Osteoporosis Formula

Enzymatic Therapy's Osteo Prime Forte

Dose: Take daily as directed, with meals.

Antioxidants

It is now widely accepted by science that upward of eighty disease processes—from diabetes, heart disease, and cancer to wrinkles, allergies, and general aging—are directly related to what is called *free radical* damage. We make free radicals in the body as part of our normal living process—they are used by our immune system to destroy bacteria and viruses—but if made in excess or if unchecked by antioxidants, they can accelerate aging and create disease. Environmental pollution, smoking, synthetic chemicals, and ultraviolet radiation all create free radicals and add to our need for increased antioxidant protection.

Antioxidants have a relationship with each other that is regenerative—they keep each other active longer—so it is best to take a broad-spectrum antioxidant formula that contains traditionally recognized antioxidants like vitamins C, E, beta-carotene and selenium, as well as a mixture of recently recognized important phytochemicals like *sulphorphane,* from broccoli; *lycopene,* from tomatoes; *proanthocyanidins,* from grapes; and *bioflavonoids,* from various sources. Recently, a few studies have claimed that beta-carotene, in supplemental form is not effective, and one study even raised the question of its possibly being dangerous. These studies are out of sync with the vast majority of world research, which shows that beta-carotene, even in supplemental form, has positive health benefits. The negative studies point out that it is futile to give a synthetic version of a real substance in small doses to high-risk populations and expect miraculous health benefits because this is completely unrealistic.

Brands we recommend:

Prevail's Antioxidant Formula
RxVitamins' The Antioxidant Formula
Enzymatic Therapy's Doctor's Choice Antioxidant
Naturally Vitamins': Maxi Flav or MaxiZzap
Tyler Encapsulation's Cyto-Redoxin or Oxyperm
Pycnogenol®—vaious brands

Dose: Take daily as directed on the label, with meals.

Essential Fatty Acids (EFAs)

Essential fatty acids protect your arteries, can help maintain an ideal weight, can decrease tumor growth, can decrease pain, and can normalize your hormones. We don't get enough of these good oils and often instead get too many harmful fats and oils. You get small amounts of EFAs in your daily diet, and more significant quantities in cold-water fish like tuna or salmon. The most reliable vegetarian source is flaxseed. Flaxseed provides benefits from its omega-3 oils, vitamin E, lecithin (which helps emulsify fats), phytosterols, and high amounts of lignans, which can be converted into protective estrogenic substances; lignans also provide powerful antioxidant properties. You can find flaxseed in health food stores, generally in the seeds and nuts section. You can buy them by the pound, prepackaged, or in powder or oil form. One way to use them very effectively is to grind fresh seeds and spinkle a tablespoon or so a day on soups, salads, casseroles, or smoothies. In this way you get the benefit of both the lignan and the essential fatty acid in the fresh seed. Pumpkin, borage, sunflower, hazelnut, and evening primrose oils also contain varying amounts of EFAs. We recommend products that are organic and have a combination of EFAs to provide you with broad-spectrum health benefits.

Brands we recommend:

Omega Nutrition's Essential Balance, Essential Balance Jr., or Flax Borage combo
Arrowhead Mill's Essential Balance
Enzymatic Therapy's Doctor's Choice Flax Oil Plus
Solgar's MaxEPA
Cardinova's Eskimo 3
Barlean's Flax/Borage
Naturally Vitamins' Omega Marine Lipids

Dose: Take two to three capsules two times per day with meals or one teaspoon to one tablespoon two times per day with meals.

Green Super Foods

There is no category of food supplement that is as broad in its life-supporting benefits as the green super foods. Included in this group of foods are *chlorella* (green microalgae), *spirulina* (blue-green algae), *wheat, barley,* and *alfalfa* grasses. Spirulina and chlorella are said to be the first life forms found on the planet over three and a half billion years ago. They are simple single-cell algaes. With today's technologies, these simple plants are grown in controlled environments for purity and quality. They are available in health food stores and can be the perfect complement to your multivitamin and mineral supplements. They can be taken in powder, capsule, or tablet form. They are reported to help regulate your hunger, normalize blood sugar, decrease inflammation, and provide powerful phytochemical protection for everything from heart disease to cancer to premature aging.

Chlorella. Chlorella is the most studied natural food in the world and is the second-largest-selling health food in Japan, where it is classified as a *functional food.* This category of food is recognized by the Japanese government as having important therapeutic value, yet it is not a drug. It is a complete food with over twenty bio-available vitamins and minerals. It contains over 60 percent complete digestible protein and nineteen naturally occurring amino acids, including all the eight essential amino acids. It has been shown to promote cellular reproduction, reduce cholesterol, and increase hemoglobin levels. Ingestion of its fibrous cell wall (cellulose) improves digestion and promotes the growth of beneficial intestinal flora, in addition to helping eliminate dangerous toxins from your body.

Spirulina. Spirulina is one of nature's most nutrient-dense foods. Besides being a complete source of quality vegetable protein at levels over 60 percent, it contains over a dozen valuable phytochemicals, including levels of beta-carotene ten times those found in carrots. Meat protein contains high saturated fat, uric acid, red blood cells, no fiber, gristle, and, frequently, antibiotic residue. Spirulina protein contains no saturated fats, only essential fatty acids. It contains a vast array of antioxidants, B vitamins, fiber, and chlorophyll and other phytochemicals needed to prevent disease. It provides an easy-to-digest protein without any of the drawbacks of meat. It also contains 350 percent more potassium than rice and 300 percent more iron than red meat. Spirulina is very low in fat and is about 15 to 25 percent carbohydrate. It is a great resource for long-term energy and stamina as well as stable blood sugar levels. And it curbs your appetite naturally.

Cereal grasses. Back in the 1930s, before vitamin pills became available, people took tablets of dehydrated grasses like barley, wheat, or alfalfa to correct nutritional deficiencies. Since then, the research on the value and health benefits of cereal grasses has progressed. These grasses are a highly nutritious and staple food with nutritional contents that resemble those of organic green leafy vegetables. For example, a few tablets can give you the nutritional and phytochemical equivalent of a healthy green salad. Like green vegetables, these grasses contain significant amounts of beta-carotene, iron, calcium, folic acid, and vitamin C, as well as many other trace elements. However, unlike other vegetables, wheat, barley, and alfalfa grasses contain all of the essential amino acids in balanced and usable proportions.

The products we are recommending are grown in organic soils for several hundred days; their roots grow deep and concentrate myriad essential elements from the earth. The grass is then harvested and prepared in various forms, like powder, tablets, and capsules. While drinking fresh-squeezed wheat grass from a health food store has good health benefits, it is grown on a flat and doesn't have the full extent of the benefits of wheat grass grown in soil.

All the green super foods are valuable sources of *chlorophyll.* Chlorophyll is a known infection fighter, detoxifier, and blood builder and is now being studied by the National Cancer Institute for its potential role in protection against cancer. Its benefits include its ability to remove toxic pesticides and drug residues from your system, as well as to bind with radioactive material and remove it from your body.

We recommend that you use combination products of the green super foods—both *land based* and *aquatic*—to get maximum benefits from their unique properties. If you can't always eat at least five servings of fresh fruits and vegetables a day, green super foods are one sure way to get all the nutrition and health benefits that you can get from vegetables.

Brands we recommend:

Nature's Balance Chlorella
Green Foods' Green Magma
Orange Peel Enterprises' Greens +
Pines International—all of their greens products
Microlight's Nutrejuva
Futurebiotics' Vital Greens or Alfalfa-Barley-Chlorella
Solgar's Greens 'N More

Dose: Take as directed.

The following suggestions are optional but very effective.

Digestive Supplements

Although it's been said, "You are what you eat," the truth is more that you are what you absorb and utilize from your food. Digestive enzymes are responsible for breaking down our food into readily available nutrients for the body to utilize more efficiently. Because of aging, stress, poor diet, environmental factors, and drugs, our digestive strength and capacity diminishes. Women who experience problems with their digestion and resort to frequent antacids are certainly not getting the full benefit of nutrients and phytosterols for hormonal balancing. In addition, poor digestion can interfere with the absorption of our recommended hormonal products. Taking digestive supplements is a way to ensure that you are getting the most from your meals. They are nontoxic and safe for long-term use, and they can help strengthen your digestive system. There is no standardization of these types of products as of this writing, so for the best effects we suggest you choose from the brands below.

Brands we recommend:

Prevail's Vitase Digestive Enzyme
Rainbow Light's Advance Enzyme System
Futurebiotics' Vegetarian Enzyme Complex
Tyler Encapsulations' Similase
Naturally Vitamins' Wobenzym

Dose: Two to four capsules at the beginning of each meal help to ensure a broad range of efficient digestion for optimal absorption.

Take plant enzymes for one to two months, then let your experience guide you on whether to continue or stop. The benefits also include less gas, more regular bowel movements, less indigestion, fewer food allergies, and, often, more energy.

Caution: If you have an ulcer or a pre-ulcerous condition like chronic gastritis, with symptons like heartburn or acid indigestion, do not take these products initially. Instead, use Prevail's Acid Ease for about two months, then gradually switch over. You should consult a health-care practitioner.

Probiotics

Several hundred different species of intestinal microorganisms (our friendly intestinal flora) live in unison with us within our bodies. They are necessary for our life in much the same way that soil organisms are needed to turn soil elements into available food for plants. When these organisms are compromised, then pathogenic, or disease-causing, organisms can take up residence and literally alter our internal environments, setting the stage for illness.

Poor dietary habits, smoking, stress, chlorinated water, alcohol, aging, antibiotics and many other drugs all contribute to a decrease in your necessary friendly flora. One way to help improve their quality and quantity is to eat natural, whole, organic foods. They are rich in the fiber and nutrients that support flora growth. Fermented foods like yogurt, sauerkraut, and miso also replenish and support your intestinal health. But the fastest way to jump-start an improved intestinal environment is to supplement these organisms with a probiotic product. The word "probiotic" means pro life. These products contain many different species of healthy flora like *acidophilus* and *bifidus,* plus a food product called FOS (fructooligosaccharides). FOS is a naturally occurring carbohydrate found in foods like onions and asparagus and helps feed the friendly flora as well as helping to reestablish their colonization in your intestines.

If you suffer from digestive problems, you should definitely consider these supplements. In fact, most everyone will benefit from and improve their health by supplementing their diet intermittently with probiotics.

Products we recommend:

Prevail's Inner Ecology
RxVitamins' CDA-21
Natures' Way's Prima Dolphilus

Natren's Healthy Trinity
Ethical Nutrients' Intestinal Care
Naturally Vitamins' Fructodophilus or Super Acidophilus

Dose: Take the recommended dose two times per day between meals, with water, either half an hour before your meal or one to two hours after eating. We recommend doing this for several months to start, then reintroducing one or two bottles every three months.

Adaptogens

Adaptogens are herbal substances that fit specific criteria for helping the body to "adapt" to stresses, whether internal or external. Although there are no direct studies for their use for menopausal symptoms, they can be very helpful to your overall well-being. The first natural substance to be termed an adaptogen was Panax ginseng in the 1940s. The Chinese have extolled its virtues for thousands of years. Other recognized adaptogens now include Siberian ginseng, suma, schizandra, astragalus, and reishi mushroom. Adaptogens by their very nature work nonspecifically—that is, they affect your endocrine, nervous, cardiovascular, reproductive, and musculoskeletal systems to provide better functioning and balance. Also, by definition, they must be harmless and nontoxic and able to be used long term. Documented benefits are increased mental alertness and work productivity. They are widely utilized by athletes to increase stamina and endurance and thus improve athletic performance.

Though you can experience significant benefits in energy and alertness right from the start, adaptogens yield even more rewards cumulatively. The longer you take them, the better you feel.

Brands we recommend:

Enzymatic Therapy's Siberian Ginseng
Zand's Active Herbal
Futurebiotics' Reishi Mushroom
Rainbow Light's East Earth Herbs

Dose: Take the amount directed in the morning. You can repeat in the afternoon when you need an extra lift or before a workout. In general, it's best not to use at night.

Care of the Face

From Cleopatra to Cher, women have been using plants to enhance the quality of their skin. The Duchess of Windsor was reputed to have said something to the effect that when a woman gets older she can cover up below the neck, but she must never forget the care of the face. We're obviously not advocating this approach, but it speaks to a truth about female beauty and a youthful presentation. The face is that which you show to the world, and taking care of it *naturally*—without resorting to surgical intervention—is what we are addressing here.

There are many fine plant preparations that will enhance the quality of your skin, but we single out alpha-hydroxy acids, or natural fruit-sugar acids, for their particular effectiveness. They gently exfoliate the top dead layer of the skin, leading to a more youthful, fresher complexion. They are helpful in lightening brown spots and smoothing out fine wrinkles and skin roughness and irregularities and reducing large pores.

Over-the-counter products that contain alpha-hydroxy acids don't clearly show how much is in their preparations. To make sure of what you're getting, a dermatologist or facialist can make up a product to suit you. In most cases, you need an 8 to 10 percent concentration to produce results, but many over-the-counter products are just 2 to 3 percent. You should get a slight tingling reaction to know it is working; then you can increase the strength as your skin adapts.

Prima Facie makes a nasturtium cream that contains a mixture of fruit acids and progesterone and is very effective. Creams with a progesterone content have been shown to be excellent moisturizers.

You might also want to consider organic cosmetic products, which are free of harmful additives.

Brands we recommend:

Aubrey Organics	800-282-7394
Zia Cosmetics	800-334-7546
AnnMarie Borlind products	
Educated Beauty	800-323-8423
Prima Facie	800-900-9265 (Canada)
	800-413-2242 (U.S.)

14

TAKING CARE OF YOUR BONES

There is no *single* treatment for either the prevention or reversal of osteoporosis. Prevention starts with a healthy plant-based diet and exercise, and includes avoidance of proprietary drugs, such as synthetic cortisone, which leech bone mass. Once osteoporosis has set in, it *can* be reversed, but it's important to work on every front—with diet, exercise, supplementation, and, depending on the severity of the symptoms, the use of "the naturals."

A Visit to the Doctor

You're a forty-five-plus woman and you finally decide (after a good long time with your head in the sand) to visit your internist or gynecologist in the hope that osteoporosis has nothing to do with the still young and vibrant you.

Tests ordered for you confirm either bone loss or the possibility of it in the near future. Another test shows your estrogen levels to be diminishing, and you may or may not have begun to have menopausal symptoms. *But I'm in the prime of my life! Old ladies aren't sexy!* And you immediately project yourself as five inches shorter, with a spine like a bent spoon, sitting on a park bench talking about all your *other* ailments.

Your chances for developing osteoporosis are greatly increased if you are light-skinned and fair-haired, if you have a family history of the disease, if you are small and thin, if you've never been pregnant, if you've had a hysterectomy or oophorectomy (removal of the ovaries), and on and on. The list is extensive and mind-numbing. To top it off, we now know that bone loss starts early in life, with half of spinal bone loss occurring before menopause. The average untreated woman loses four inches in height during her lifetime. And most doctors believe that what you've already lost cannot be replaced. Talk about depressing.

Osteoporosis is epidemic in this country in women over the age of sixty, and is said to be pandemic if you live long enough. One third of all women in the United States sixty and older have spinal compression fractures. These fractures can cause varying degrees of pain, spinal deformations, and height loss. They may cause such symptoms as loss of appetite, heartburn, and bloating, as well as difficulty in breathing, although a direct association between these symptoms and osteoporosis may be a difficult diagnosis to make.[1] More than 25 million Americans, primarily women, are high-risk candidates for developing osteoporosis. The World Health Organization has declared osteoporosis the second-largest health risk for women after heart disease. It is responsible for over a million and a half bone fractures a year.[2]

When you think of bone, you most likely think of a skeleton, which is, of course, dead. And hard and brittle. But everything we think we know about bones from looking at skeletons is completely off base. They are not just dead sticks inside your skin. Bones are living tissue. They have blood vessels and nerves. They are constantly growing. They live and breathe and change from moment to moment.

Cosmonauts returning from the *Soyuz 34* space flight had to be taken off the spacecraft on stretchers because, after 175 days in space, their muscles and bones had deteriorated to the point at which they were unable to stand. Why did this happen? Because, in large measure, not enough stress was put on their bones in the microgravity of space flight. Bones are *dynamic.* And very *efficient.* Being weightless, the cosmonauts' bodies immediately said, "Why do I need these heavy bones if I'm not using them?" and adjusted accordingly. In the body's infinite wisdom, it adapts quickly to changing needs. The cosmonauts' bodies took calcium and other minerals from their bones and within hours started eliminating it, mostly through urine. The result: When they returned to earth, their bones would not support them.

The human body reacts *dynamically,* wanting to establish an equilibrium in every situation in which it finds itself. It monitors automatically and adjusts accordingly. The bottom line is: If you don't use it, you lose it.

Besides giving your body *structure* and *support,* your bones function as a *storage depot,* which saves up the material you need to correct shortages or deficiencies elsewhere in your body. For example, your blood must always be in a state of slight alkalinity. As soon as your blood becomes too acidic, a condition that can be brought on by poor diet or stress, the minerals in your bones—primarily calcium and magnesium—are pulled from your "storage depot" to act as buffers and correct the situation. Before you can say *osteoporosis,* calcium and other minerals are depleted from your bone stores, and when finished with their job, are urinated out—gone, but not forgotten. What is taken out must be replaced, but, if you are making more withdrawals than deposits, you will end up with the dreaded osteoporosis.

In the simplest possible terms, osteoporosis—which means "porous bones"—is a depletion of the mineral components of bone. The bones begin to lose their ability to withstand pressure, hence pathological fractures. Can you imagine a worse old age than being in persistent and intractable pain—because advanced osteoporosis is *very* painful—and trying to move on bones that don't support you, that can shear or crack with the slightest amount of pressure? This enormous suffering is completely avoidable.

Why Do We Get Osteoporosis?

Most Western women on a Western diet—if they live long enough—will get this disease. But in Asia, the incidence of osteoporosis among women is almost nonexistent. Women in Asian countries can live to a very old age without any signs of bone degeneration.

How can this be? Well, we know that there are significant dietary differences between Asian and Western women. As already discussed in chapter 4, besides an absence of processed food in their diets, Asian women eat much less protein and more vegetables and grains, affording them more minerals and nutrients. They eat plant foods high in phytosterols, such as tofu, miso, and other soy products; legumes (beans); and other plants and herbs. This diet seems to protect them from other menopausal symptoms as well.

Rural Asian women generally don't concern themselves with bone loss, in good measure because exercise is an integral part of their daily lives. Their demanding way of life provides all the exercise they need to give their bones the stress necessary to keep them strong and healthy. For example, they walk distances to get their water, often balancing jugs on their heads. They don't have many technological or electrical luxuries that help to create our sedentary lifestyles.

And these rural women certainly don't go around popping calcium pills. In fact, their average daily dietary calcium consumption is estimated at around 300 milligrams. As we've discussed briefly earlier, several studies have shown that when these women become "Westernized"—eating processed foods, a diet high in protein, fat, and sugar, and adopting a lifestyle without the benefits of regular exercise—they, too, begin to suffer typical menopausal symptoms at the same rate as modern Western women. If they return to their native cultures and resume their former way of life, the osteoporosis risk factor goes back to what it was.[3]

Pollution, pesticides, intentional additives, and hidden contaminants in food, and the increasing stress of life, all play havoc with your poor put-upon bones. Just think about the stress you bring into play by juggling career and family life. Simple common sense can tell us it is our present diet/lifestyle/environment that leads to the "inevitable" loss of bone mass and the completely preventable, crippling killer (mainly of women) called osteoporosis.

But now you know. And knowledge is power. Armed with this new understanding, you can fight back and take charge of the health of your bones.

The Standard Prescription

Mostly likely you will be sent home with the standard medical prescription: Premarin, or another of the estrogen replacement therapy (ERT) drugs; the exhortation to get 1,000 to 1,500 milligrams of calcium a day; and perhaps the suggestion that you should exercise.

You are told to take the Premarin for the rest of your life. (You're also told that low estrogen levels can make you vulnerable to heart disease, another reason for which you should take Premarin, which darkens your mood even more.) And most likely, if you have an intact uterus, you are also told to take Provera, which is to protect you from ovarian cancer, for which you are now at greater risk by taking the Premarin.

Estrogen and Bone Loss

Although the use of the common ERT drugs has been shown to *slow bone loss in women, it does not arrest it.* Picture what goes on in your bones this way: A pair of switches regulate business. One switch gets *rid of excess minerals* (osteoclasts), and one switch *builds bone density* (osteoblasts). Estrogen works on the switch that gets rid of excess minerals by slowing down the *rate of loss.* It's a little like putting gum on a leaky faucet. You've slowed down the drip, but the faucet will continue to leak, albeit at a slower rate.

Slowing down bone loss is in no way the same as building bone mass. And not only does the use of estrogen for osteoporosis have only a partial effect, but what effect it does have is not necessarily permanent. One group of researchers found that within four years of discontinuing ERT, there was no detectable difference in bone mineral content between women who had never taken the drug and those who began treatment but gave it up. Others studies have shown that six years into menopause, ERT may stop being effective.[4]

Does this justify putting your health at serious risk for a possible—but not established—benefit? We think you would agree that the answer is no. Especially when we have a far better and more complete answer without the risk.

Progesterone for Bones

Recent studies have pointed to the importance of progesterone in building bone.

John Lee, M.D., a prolific researcher in this subject, has conducted patient studies on the power of progesterone in building bone mass and has published his findings in leading medical journals and in *What Your Doctor May* Not *Tell You About Menopause* (Warner Books, 1996).[5]

The most significant studies to date on progesterone for bone loss have been done by Dr. Jerilynn Prior of the University of British Columbia. Her work with both humans and animals has very clearly shown that not only can progesterone arrest bone loss, it can do something that estrogen can't: It can actually create *new* bone formation.[6] *Progesterone* works on the switches that build bone mass. Progesterone is invited in and turns on the bone-building process. In addition, it sends a message to the other switch to stop any bone loss.

Despite this clear evidence of the importance of progesterone to bone formation, very little attention has been given to it by the medical establishment. Dr. William Regelson, a leading researcher in hormones and the author of *The Super-Hormone Promise,* flatly states, "Given the fact that 25 percent of all women are at risk of developing osteoporosis, I think it is unconscionable that progesterone's role in this disease has been neglected."[7]

While *progestins* can have some of the benefits of progesterone on bone remineralization, they also have serious side effects, which is not true of natural progesterone. The 1995 PEPI study confirmed this.

Estriol for Bone

In three very important new studies, estriol (E3) has been shown to prevent bone loss in postmenopausal women. As we believe the use of estriol (E3) is a safer alternative for long term therapy to estrogen regimens of estrone (E1) and estradiol (E2), this is very good news for women.[i]

---

[i] H. Minaguchi, et al. Effect of estriol on bone loss in postmemopausal Japanese women: a multicenter prospective open study. *J. Obstet Gynaecol Res,* 1996 Jun 22(3):259–65.

M. Nozaki, et al. Usefulness of estriol for the treatment of bone loss in postmenopausal women. *Acta Obstetrica et Gynaecologica Japonica,* 1996 Feb 48(2): 83–8.

A. Nishibe, et al. Effect of estriol and bone mineral density of lumbar vertebrae in elderly and postmemopausal women. *Japanese Journal of Geriatrics,* 1996 May, 33(5): 353–9.

Testosterone and DHEA (Dehydroepioandosterone) for Bone

New findings are beginning to show the role of testosterone in the building of bone. While testosterone is predominantly a male hormone, it is present in a woman in smaller amounts and has important physiologic effects. One third of your testosterone is made in your ovaries.

Testosterone has been labeled the "feel good" hormone, as it increases energy and libido. In very large doses it has masculinizing effects. Besides these effects, like progesterone, it has a bone-building capacity for both men and women. Interestingly enough, men who have low levels of testosterone have a higher incidence of osteoporosis.[8]

Bone density and serum DHEA levels both decline with advancing years. Even though there is no direct correlation established as of yet, there is evidence that aging alone cannot explain the relationship between lower DHEA and declining bone mass. In a study conducted on Belgian women, a significant correlation was established between bone mineral content and DHEA levels. This held true even after correcting for the effects of age.[9]

In another study it was shown that although DHEA levels declined with age in two groups of women, those who had osteoporosis and those of a similar age without osteoporosis, those with osteoporosis had the lower levels of DHEA at all ages.[10] Experiments done almost two decades ago showed plasma levels of DHEA (DHEA-s) to be markedly lower in post-menopausal osteoporotic women than in matched controls.

In a study of post-menopausal women, administering DHEA increased serum levels of both testosterone and estrogen.[11] Administration of DHEA to ovariectomized rats significantly increased bone mineral density.[12]

DHEA may be important in the treatment and prevention of osteoporosis in several ways. It does this by stimulating bone formation and calcium absorption. DHEA also appears to have a by-product that can adhere to estrogen receptors and thereby inhibit bone resorption.

Fosamax

As of this writing, the most widely touted proprietary drug for the treatment of osteoporosis is called Fosamax, introduced in 1994.

Preliminary studies show that it can increase bone mass, but we believe use of it should be approached with flashing red caution lights. Similar to preceding drugs, such as Didronel, that stop bone resorption, Fosamax is a substance that is foreign to your body and doesn't exist anywhere in nature, and although there is evidence that it does make bone, the bone that it makes is not exactly the same as normal human bone. It is more brittle—which could lead to a greater possibility of bone fractures in women.

Of great concern to us is that the use of Fosamax is recommended for life; once you start, you shouldn't stop, and the bone mineral crystal that is formed is immovable. This brings up innumerable concerns about the bone's ability to function naturally or even heal itself. In addition, there have been no long-term studies about using this foreign substance for a lengthy period of time.

Of even greater concern is a recent 1996 study in *The New England Journal of Medicine* that called attention to an alarming number of women who suffered serious damage to their esophagi when using Fosamax. If the drug is not taken with a sufficient amount of water, complications can result. The drug company is now recommending that patients remain sitting or standing for at least half an hour after taking the drug and that they not lie down immediately after. We recommend staying away from drugs with such dangerous side effects.[13]

Calcium Alone Is Not Enough

As we've said, Asian women only get the equivalent of 300 milligrams of calcium in their daily diets, yet live to ripe old ages without evidence of osteoporosis. Is calcium important for your bones? Of course. *Very important.* Calcium adds structure and rigidity to bone. But just as your car needs gas to run, it also needs transmission fluid, steering fluid, and other essentials. These other elements may be needed in smaller amounts, but without them, your car won't run.

For example, you need:

Magnesium. Magnesium is necessary to build bone. Not only does magnesium increase the bone's ability to absorb calcium, it has been reported that even a mild magnesium deficiency is a leading risk factor in the development of osteoporosis. Magnesium enhances the absorption and utilization of calcium, activates vitamin D, and helps with the proper functions of the bone-related hormones parathyroid and calcitonin. Post-menopausal osteoporosis is primarily a demineralization process involving the weight-bearing, or trabecular, bones—that is, the spine, the femur, and the hip joint. Recent studies indicated that oral supplementation daily with 600 milligrams of magnesium and only 500 milligrams of calcium may not only help prevent bone loss but may increase bone re-mineralization of these weight-bearing bones.[14] In one study with daily dosages between 600 and 1,000 milligrams of magnesium and 500 milligrams of calcium being administered to women for one year it was observed that the women had an 11 percent increase in bone density.

Unfortunately, many of the studies that show that calcium supplementation in daily amounts of 1,000 to 1,500 milligrams may increase the bone mineral density of corticol bone (the non-weight-bearing bones like your wrist and arm) but is not significantly effective at increasing the re-mineralization of the all-important trabecular bones. The traditional thinking that advocates calcium alone for bones needs to be broadened to include important minerals like magnesium.

Studies have shown that taking the proper ratio of minerals, as we recommend in our plan, have not only stopped bone loss but have restored both trabecular and corticol bone tissue.

Vitamin D. Vitamin D is essential to calcium absorption and bone mineralization. Calcium and vitamin D relate to each other like a locked door and key: Vitamin D is the "key" that unlocks the door, allowing calcium to leave the intestine and enter the bloodstream. Vitamin D is the body's primary regulator of calcium absorption. Even small amounts of vitamin D have been shown to dramatically increase calcium absorption and significantly slow the rate of bone loss.

Vitamin K. It helps maintain *osteocalcin*, a hormone necessary for bone mineralization. Vitamin K enables osteocalcin to attract and hold calcium within the bone. Studies show that vitamin K supplementation can significantly reduce bone loss in osteoporotic women.[15]

Boron. Boron is an ultra-trace mineral, meaning that you need very little of it, but it is still *essential* for optimal calcium metabolism. This mineral helps activate both vitamin D and estrogen, thus enhancing their individual protective effects. Deficiencies in boron can result in reduced blood levels of ionized calcium and calcitonin. And a magnesium deficiency will actually increase your need for boron.

Manganese. The basketball superstar Bill Walton suffered from numerous unexplained fractures and was diagnosed with osteoporosis. Tests showed that he had plenty of calcium (his levels were actually high), but that he was deficient in *manganese* and the trace elements *zinc* and *copper.* Walton's diet was changed, he started taking mineral supplements, and within six weeks he was back playing basketball.

Phosphorus. Although a much needed component of bone, *too much* phosphorus in the diet—from meat and carbonated sodas, among many other sources—actually accelerates the osteoporosis process.

The one-note emphasis on *calcium, calcium, calcium* as the fixer of bone problems has had the effect of deflecting attention from the absolute necessity of other minerals and nutrients in building strong bone. And if you're not deficient in calcium and you are taking 1,500 milligrams of calcium a day, you can actually be making an osteoporosis problem worse. Too much calcium can interfere with the absorption of manganese—this was true for Bill Walton—and excess calcium may very well head for your eyes, your arteries, and your brain—everywhere but where you want it to go.

The bottom line is that although calcium is essential, it is not the *only* element you need for healthy bones. You need a *balance* of nutrients from diet and supplementation, combined with exercise, to ensure that you are doing right by your bones.

The Right Exercise

If you are swimming once a week as your only exercise, that is a start, but you are not doing enough for your bones. It is *weight-bearing and resistance exercise* that puts the demand on your body that will strengthen your bones. Remember, your bones are *dynamic.* If you are just sitting around all day on your butt, your bones will adjust very efficiently to your sedentary state.

But once the good stress of exercise is put on your bones, they will respond happily and quickly. This is why we can't emphasize enough that for the health of your bones, *exercise is not optional.*

In chapter 15 we are going to make a strong case for strength training with weights as the best overall exercise regime. Until recently, upper-body strength has been seriously neglected as part of a woman's conditioning, but a strong upper body, flexibility, and good posture are essential factors in a youthful, sexy physique. A dowager's hump and weak arms are not loaded with sex appeal!

Don't be put off by the idea that weights are just for bodybuilders, or that you'll get *too* muscular. You'd have to work for *years* at an exhaustive pace to look like a bodybuilder, and the right training regime does *not* build excess muscle. But by weight training, you can become lean, fit, sexy, and strong. There's no reason on earth you can't be strong and fit for the whole of your life span. It is your heritage. It is in your genes. For thousands of years, women in hunter-gatherer tribes spent their days walking long distances to collect food, digging roots and tubers, hauling heavy loads of firewood and water, often while carrying a young child, and then having plenty of energy left over to dance vigorously for hours. Unlike what we see in contemporary society, these early ancestors maintained both cardiovascular and musculoskeletal fitness for the whole of their life spans. There's no reason why you can't do the same.

The Natural Woman Plan Summary

Take an osteoporosis test as described in chapter 10. Depending on what the test reveals and what level of intervention you decide is needed, follow the plan for:

Exercise
Dietary supplements and herbal formulas
Progesterone, if needed
Tri-est with progesterone, if needed
Testosterone, depending on need and therapeutic choice
DHEA, depending on need and therapeutic choice

15

AN IDEAL WAY TO EXERCISE

A Quiz

What can . . .

Decrease your risk of breast cancer by 50 percent?
Protect you against heart disease?
Increase your "good" cholesterol (HDL) and lower "bad" cholesterol (LDL)?
Increase the number of red and white blood cells?
Increase your blood circulation?
Lower your blood pressure?
Improve your memory?
Increase your bone density, strength, and resiliency?
Decrease the amount of stress hormones in your body?
Smooth and plump up your skin?
Make you look and feel younger?

A new wonder drug?

Not at all. Just plain old exercise. That's right. *Exercise.* Everything we've listed above is backed up with numerous scientific studies.

We have a tendency to think of exercise as a *cosmetic,* something that will fix our flabby thighs and tuck in our stomachs—just improving the outer look of the package. But exercise is an important *instrument* of your health. It not only tones up your muscles, but works on your whole anatomy. It works in concert with your metabolism for the better handling of nutrients: Exercise added to nutrients *upgrades* their effectiveness and efficiency. In other words, one plus one equals three.

And lack of exercise parallels every aspect of aging.

We are made up of muscles and bones, which, in turn, provide structure and movement, and in order for these components to maintain their vitality, they must be *moved.* When you wake up in the morning, you brush your teeth and gums to keep them healthy and prevent decay. In the same way, you should consider *movement* as preventive care for your body. You must keep the component parts "well oiled" and "primed." And when you don't move, these component parts lose their viability, and the aging process is accelerated—not just in your muscles and bones but in all the organs of your body. You were born to dance!

According to one study, women of childbearing age who exercise four or more hours per week can halve their risk of breast cancer before menopause.[1] Exercise is directly linked to your hormonal health.

The Superior Benefits of Strength Training

The reason we will be emphasizing strength (or weight) training over other forms of exercise in this book is because it is the *quickest* in terms of visible results, health gains, and time expended. It is also the most *reliable,* and the most *measurable,* in terms of overall result, and is the only exercise that can actually *reverse* existing conditions such as loss of lean body mass and bone density.

Unfortunately, it is also the most misunderstood by women.

The use of weights evolved out of body-building competition and was definitely a guy's game at first. But over the past ten years, the use of weights for strength training for both sexes has greatly evolved and has become extremely sophisticated. When applied to women's muscles, it means using all the latest technology to tighten your ligaments and joints, thighs, tummy and tush, while improving your body composition and more quickly strengthening you. We are not talking Charles Atlas or Arnold Schwarzenegger here. You will not be adding significant or unsightly bulk. Lean, strong, and toned is the goal. And pound for pound, *muscle burns much more fat* . . . the more muscle weight you have, the more calories you burn. A pound of fat burns only four kilocalories a day. A pound of muscle burns *thirty-five to fifty kilocalories* a day. "Strength training revs up your metabolic rate, so you burn more calories whatever you are doing, even when sitting and sleeping . . . After age forty-five or so, sedentary people—and even many who do aerobic exercise—rapidly lose muscle mass and, consequently, strength . . . The lost strength largely accounts for the difficulty many elderly people have in rising from chairs, climbing stairs, and carrying groceries," says an article advocating strength training for women in *The New York Times* in 1994.[2]

Among the other established benefits of strength training:

- improved performance in other sports, like tennis, golf, and swimming
- increased flexibility
- greater endurance for both chores and recreational activity
- loss of body fat and gain of lean muscle tissue, resulting in improved body composition
- more energy and self-confidence
- a greater sense of physical and emotional well-being[3]
- increased balance and tensile strength, thereby reducing the likelihood of falling

Common Myths Women Believe About Strength/Weight Training

Myth: It will make me look bulky.

Reality: Men increase muscle size more from lifting weights because they have greater amounts of the male hormone necessary for muscle growth, so unless you're lifting heavy weights many hours a day, or taking anabolic (male) steroids (God forbid), you will not gain unfeminine bulk.

Myth: I'll gain weight.

Reality: Muscle does weigh more than fat, and you will be changing the composition of your body by decreasing fat and increasing lean mass. In fact, it is not uncommon for a woman to drop a clothing size, but not lose pounds. Muscle is more *dense* than fat. You will actually shrink in overall size—in addition to tightening and lifting, particularly your backside. Tables for the ideal weights for women are based on an unmuscled body, and you will adopt a different standard for your weight based on your overall size.

Myth: Strength training will turn my fat into muscle.

Reality: Nothing turns fat cells into muscle cells; they are two completely different types of tissues. You can, however, use the energy derived from burning fat calories to build and strengthen your muscle fibers. This is one of the reasons men are able to eat more without gaining weight. They carry more muscle, thereby burning more calories.

Myth: It'll take too much time.

Reality: You might be shocked to learn that once you have reached your goal, then just *one hour per week*, plus an additional hour and a half of some kind of cardiovascular activity, will do the trick for you. Unless, of course, your goal is to complete a marathon or enter a body-building competition. And more than any other exercise, you can see results in as little as a few weeks, as previously little-used muscle is given better definition, tone, and strength.

Myth: I'm too old for this kind of thing.

Reality: Strength training works at any age. It can get even ninety-year-olds up and out of their wheelchairs.

From *The New York Times,* August 10, 1994:

> "In just 10 weeks of a strength-training program, 50 frail men and women in their 80's and 90's were able to increase their

> weight-lifting ability by 118 percent, their walking speed by 12 percent and their stair climbing ability by 28 percent, according to a study published last month in *The New England Journal of Medicine*. . . . Impressive though these accomplishments are in stemming some of the costly and debilitating incapacities of old age, they pale in comparison with what strength training can do for younger people who want to maintain or improve physical prowess . . ."[4]

For women past forty, the benefits are huge, as they have more to gain than their younger sisters from strength training. Younger women have a greater reserve of muscle and strength beyond the amount required to maintain everyday activities, but as women get older, they get more sedentary and begin losing valuable muscle. Of course, starting early is always better than playing catch-up in later life, but even with a preexisting condition such as heart disease or arthritis, with the right program you can achieve amazing results at any age.

And *muscle* is just as important as bone density in the prevention of osteoporosis. "Bone density is only one element in these fractures [from osteoporosis]. It may be even more important to improve women's muscle strength and balance to prevent falls, which are the greatest risk factor for fractures in the elderly."[5] So says the leader of a 1994 study reported in *The Journal of the American Medical Association* on the effectiveness of strength training for menopausal and post-menopausal women. Exercise such as swimming or any form of cardiovascular exercise cannot provide the same benefits. Only strength training can reverse the consequences of osteoporosis.

Myth: I'm not athletic and have never done anything like it before.

Reality: Strength training is, in fact, ideal for those of you who are nonathletic, assuming that you don't have a preexisting condition that would preclude this kind of exercise—and there are very few such conditions. For one thing, you can work at any level. Working with weights doesn't require athletic prowess. Even a person with heart disease or arthritis can use weights with a specially tailored program—you can begin at the lowest level and slowly work your way up.

Some women are initially nervous about working with weights—they're afraid they might hurt themselves—but since the amount of weight lifted is specifically tailored to a woman's own abilities, the lifting of weights can always be manageable at any strength.

As Chris can testify: "After my last bout with illness, I emerged extremely weak and thin and seemingly muscleless—a coffee mug seemed heavy to me, that was how weak I was. I very gradually began with strength training, at first at just zero weight, for movement alone, and within three months, I was noticeably improved; in six, I was normal for my age; and in nine, stronger and 'younger' than ever."

You're Still Not Convinced

If after listening to our arguments, you still prefer other methods, then by all means use them. Some exercise is better than none at all. If you have your own ways, and it is *real exercise,* not pretend exercise—such as convincing yourself that bending down to reach into a sock drawer is exercise—then stick with it.

But what's important to remember is that you need to exercise consistently. It's *consistency,* not just appropriate *intensity,* and hopefully, enjoyment and even passion, that brings the benefits. And positive results can be addictive and self-promoting.

Where to Exercise—at the Gym or at Home

If you're an absolute beginner, we suggest starting at a gym, otherwise you might make a big investment in equipment, quit after a few stabs at it, and then have a bunch of weights gathering dust in the garage.

It's probably wiser to invest the money, at least at first, in a gym membership, as most gyms will provide free instruction with membership. Some gyms will even provide a trainer for a number of sessions for the first month of membership. If you have trouble with self-motivation, go with a friend, or a spouse.

If you can afford it, you should consider hiring a personal trainer, at least for a few sessions. It will ease your passage into a routine and will help keep you motivated. Not all trainers are expensive.

At least in the beginning, motivation and sticking to a routine past the first tries will require some effort, but after working out consistently for two months or more, many women get hooked on the benefits, and the pleasure factor kicks in. In fact, research has shown that if you can stay with your exercise program for six months, you are extremely likely to stay with it for life. So stick with it. Then if you decide you'd prefer to train at home, you will have a routine established with either weight equipment or free weights.

A Basic Strength-Training Routine

Our basic plan calls for strength training with weight machines three days a week, with aerobic/cardiovascular/stretching exercises and rest alternated: approximately forty-five minutes of weight training three times a week, plus half an hour of cardiovascular exercise two days a week, and two days of rest. Your cardiovascular activity on days when you are not strength training can be half an hour of brisk walking.

This *three hours and fifteen minutes a week* is an optimum program. Even strength training *twice* a week, plus an alternated aerobic/cardiovascular workout, can provide good benefits. For that matter, once you have reached a peak of fitness, doing your strength training once a week, along with a daily cardiovascular routine, might very well be enough to maintain your desired goal. We recommend more frequent exercise sessions, though, and find that once women have formed the habit, they generally prefer and actually enjoy the regular activity.

A version of a schedule might look like this:

Day 1
Weights
Cardio
Stretch

Day 2
Rest

Day 3
Weights
Cardio
Stretch

Day 4
Rest

Day 5
Weights
Cardio
Stretch

Day 6
Cardio

Day 7
Cardio

Exercising at the Gym

We have designed a program that you can successfully use for the long term without the need of a personal trainer. If you have never used weight machines before (or cardiovascular machines such as a treadmill or stairclimber), ask one of the qualified employees at the gym to show you their proper use. Almost all gyms should be willing to do this free of charge as part of their orientation, or at little cost. This same routine can be adapted to home weight equipment if you decide to go that route.

Our program fits two exercise personality types: those who have been exercising fairly consistently, and those who have not. Whether you are a beginner or more experienced, you should *start slowly,* consistent with your level of fitness. Too much exercise too soon can be painful and discouraging. This is one of the most common mistakes that a woman can make starting out and we strongly recommend you go lighter rather than heavier, easier rather than tougher, at first.

Strength-Training Machines

The popularity of strength training has now improved the quality of equipment available everywhere. Although there are a number of different brands of machines—such as Cybex, Nautilus, and Universal—most fitness clubs provide a standard course of weight machines. Most machines at the better gyms have a demonstration card with a drawing that will guide you in its proper use and movement. The machines you will use include:

1. leg press—for gluteals, quadriceps, and ham strings
2. leg or knee extension—for thigh or quadriceps muscles
3. leg curl/knee flexion—for backs of thighs or hamstrings
4. chest press/bench press—for chest or pectoral and arm muscles
5. upper back/compound row—for upper back and arm muscles
6. abdominal/trunk flexion—for abdominal muscles
7. lower back/back extension—for lower back muscles
8. lat pulldown or torso/arm—for the V of the back and the undersides of the upper arms
9. butterfly/pectoral—for chest and arm or pectoral muscles
10. overhead or military press—for tops of shoulders and arms
11. deltoid fly—for tops of arms and outer shoulders or deltoid muscles
12. bicep curl—for fronts of upper arms or biceps muscles
13. triceps extension—for backs of upper arms or triceps muscles

You should work up to one full circuit each workout. Depending on your fitness level, this could take up to four months. You need not do all of the machines, and can adjust for personal preference, but the above list is designed to give you a complete body workout. After you have reached the point of doing a full circuit, you can set a goal for two complete circuits. This may seem daunting, but there is in fitness training the notion of *perceived exertion.* Even if you are lifting more weights, your perceived exertion will be less because you will be in better shape and can do the lifts more easily.

Determining the Correct Weight to Lift

Here is a simple method to choose the correct weight to lift. But before beginning, make sure you have asked a qualified trainer at the gym how to use the machines correctly. Start with the lightest possible weight if you're a beginner and lift it once gently. If it feels ridiculously light, up the weight. Do it fifteen times in perfect form, no bouncing or arching of the back, focusing on the involved muscles. Was it a challenge to finish? If it was no effort at all, you need to move to the next heavier weight on your following set. If it *was* a doable challenge, great, you found your weight! If you weren't able to finish and use good form, then you need to decrease the weight.

Repetitions

You do two sets of repetitions on each machine, resting for one minute between sets. The goal is to complete the full circuit of thirteen machines in each exercise session. However, in the beginning, use your judgment about your fatigue level.

Body Awareness

Watch your form. Form is actually more important than the amount of weight lifted. The sophisticated equipment in a contemporary gym, when used with proper form, allows you to use only the muscles necessary, relaxing all others, getting the most benefit.

When and How to Increase the Weight

In order to continue to gain strength, it is important to keep challenging yourself. This means gradually moving up the amount you lift. Bradley Norris, an exercise physiologist and owner of Malibu Health & Rehabilitation, where Chris began training, suggests the following method for increasing weight:

About every four weeks or so, instead of lifting the weight fifteen times, see how many you can complete at one time. If you can do more than the fifteen with perfect form, increase the weight on your next set. While utilizing this heavier weight, you should be able to perform at least ten repetitions with perfect form. Eventually, you will be able to move to fifteen repetitions at this new weight. Then, a few weeks later, challenge yourself again and move up to the next heaviest weight.

Note: Most gyms have free-floating five-pound weight plates that you can just set on top of the weight stack. If they do not, you may have to increase a full ten pounds on upper-body machines. Don't overdo it. We'd rather you stay with a lighter weight longer than move to a too heavy weight too soon.

The Right Way to Lift

- Before beginning, learn the proper use of the machine.
- Breath *out* during exertion and *in* when returning to neutral position. Breath evenly and *don't hold your breath.* Holding your breath can cause an unnecessary rise in blood pressure.
- Go slowly. Count to two on exertion and three or four on returning to a neutral position. Lift the weight as smoothly as possible, and release it gradually so that your muscle, not the weight itself, does the work. Your form is more important than the weight you move. Don't do anything that feels wrong or harmful. You will find that some days are easier than others and you may actually want to occasionally increase or decrease your weight accordingly for daily variations in energy or strength. Our advice is to be consistent with showing up at the gym and going through your routine, adjusting your intensity as you feel necessary. Just showing up is 80 percent of the job.
- If you experience any pain, stop lifting the weight right away. However, minor muscle soreness experienced one to three days after is to be expected and is a sign that you have done some good work.
- Allow at least forty-eight hours to elapse before lifting the same muscle-group weights again. Your muscles need time between workouts to recover. The workout creates a demand for building stronger muscle fibers and support structures and systems. Your body needs time to accomplish this.

- *Focus* your mind on the muscles being used for the particular lift. Abundant research shows that mental concentration will give increased benefits. The idea is to have the mind and body aligned—synergy is the result.
- Complete a warm-up/aerobic session before lifting weights. This "warms up" the muscles and helps prevent muscle pulls, cramps, and joint damage and will maximize your workout time by immediately preparing your muscles and circulatory system for the full demands of the exercise.
- Do another set of stretches after lifting. This cooldown phase is as important as your warm-up. It helps your muscles recover more quickly by improving blood circulation. Getting a massage is a great way to do this as well, and can be a wonderful reward.

Keep a Record of Your Workouts

Whether working out at a gym or at home, make a chart of your program and then keep track of your progress. It will help you determine any changes that need to be made and—no small matter—give you a great sense of accomplishment as you continue to gain strength and tone and shape your body.

A Typical Workout in the Gym

- *Warm-up*—five to ten minutes. On the bicycle, stairclimber, or treadmill, or an aerobic dance routine. The purpose of the warm-up is to gradually introduce your heart, lungs, and circulation to the idea of exercise and create internal heat to promote better functioning.
- *Stretching*—five minutes. Follow the series of stretches on pages 189 to 195. Do not overstretch or bounce "cold" muscles. Hold for twenty seconds, while breathing and visualizing the muscles lengthening. Keep a steady body position, hold the muscle in the stretch, and don't bounce. Bouncing causes muscles to contract and shorten instead of lengthen. The purpose of stretching is to allow full range of motion in the joints and to prevent muscle shortening and injury.
- *Your weight routine*—approximately thirty minutes.

- *Cooldown*—three to five minutes. Back on the bicycle or stair-climber or treadmill. The cooldown is intended to ease your circulation and heart back to their regular rates. Then stretch again if you have time.

Exercising at Home

If you feel you would prefer to exercise at home, the same components of strength training apply as in the gym. Keeping yourself motivated is the biggest challenge when exercising at home. Your best bet is to designate a specific time when you are in "your gym" and stick to it. You can train on either weight equipment designed for use in the home (Universal, Soloflex), in which case you would follow the routine we designed for the gym, or by using hand-held free weights (also called dumbbells—or maybe they should be called "smartbells"), available at most fitness equipment stores.

The free-weight program we have designed requires *three sets* of free weights at three different weights—light, medium, and heavy—a total of six free weights.

Small Frame/Poor or Fair Strength

Light	Medium	Heavy
3 lbs.	5 lbs.	8 lbs.

Medium or Large Frame/Good Strength

Light	Medium	Heavy
5 lbs.	8 lbs.	10 lbs.

The Home Strength-Training Program

In each exercise session, you will do a full set of the following. Determine the weight with which you can do twelve to fifteen repetitions. Work up to two or three sets of twelve to fifteen repetitions. Start slowly and use your common sense about your limits.

1. modified push-up (no weights)—for chest and arm muscles
2. lunges or stairs (no weights)

3. bent lateral row (light weights)—for back (rhomboid) and latissimus dorsi
4. abdominal crunch (no weights)—for abdominals. As you improve you can work up to thirty repetitions per set.
5. pectoral fly (medium weights)—for chest muscles (pectorals)
6. leg lift (both legs in three positions; two- to four-pound ankle weights can be added)—for hip muscles
7. deltoid fly (medium weights)—for upper arms (deltoids)
8. abdominal crunch—second set
9. upright row (medium weights)—for shoulders (trapezius)
10. biceps curl (medium to heavy dumbbells)—for fronts of upper arms (biceps)
11. triceps extension (medium weights)—for backs of upper arms (triceps)

Complete two sets of twelve to fifteen repetitions for each exercise at the suitable weight.

After four weeks, follow the same guidelines for weight increases in the exercising-in-the-gym section. If you ultimately have to go to the store for heavier weights, well, good for you.

The Cardiovascular/Aerobic Component

Ideally, your routine includes some form of "aerobic" exercise at least three times a week. Aerobic means "with oxygen," which further means you need to place your heart rate in a "target heart-rate zone," or THR, and remain in this zone for fifteen to forty minutes continuously. There are two ways to monitor your heart rate: the rule-of-thumb way, or actually taking your pulse during your workout. For example, if when using the treadmill, you are still looking at your nail polish, you are probably not working hard enough. If you are breathing hard and can't talk, then you are over your THR, but if you feel yourself working up a sweat but can still talk, then you are closing in on the right zone. After you have been working out for a few months, you can use your intuition to focus you on the right rhythm and duration.

Don't be afraid to work up a sweat. Indeed, please sweat. This is what shows that you are burning those calories and getting all the benefits exercise can offer. It may not seem ladylike to some, but it can be very satisfying and purifying, not to mention beautifying. You will actually find yourself looking forward to working up a good sweat. But if at any time you feel faint or dizzy, stop. Aerobic exercise can include walking the treadmill, stair climbing on a machine or real stairs, fast walking, jogging, cycling, or aerobic dance.

Age Range	Target Heart-Rate Zone (THR)
40 to 45	110 to 140 beats per minute
46 to 50	105 to 135 beats per minute
51 to 55	100 to 130 beats per minute
56 to 60	100 to 125 beats per minute

Don't Forget to Stretch

Stretching seems to be the easiest part of a training program to overlook, but it is very important. It helps extend your range of motion and is what is going to protect you from injury. It can also be the most enjoyable part of your routine, as good stretches can be very satisfying stress reducers. Ideally, each exercise session can start and end with a few stretches that can help protect your muscles, improve your joints, and increase your flexibility, while decreasing potential soreness. Remember: Youth is flexible, while old age is often inflexible and brittle. Hold each stretch for about twenty seconds.

Stretches

1. elbow reach—for the shoulders and back
2. door pull—for the shoulders and back
3. clasped hands—for the shoulders and back
4. chest row—for the back and chest
5. cobra—for the back and chest
6. feet together—for the inner thighs
7. double knee hold—for the lower back and legs
8. one knee hold—for the lower back and legs
9. knee over trunk—for the lower back

10. hurdler's stretch—for the back, pelvis, hamstrings, and inner thighs
11. runner's start—for the pelvis and legs
12. praying mantis—for the hamstrings
13. wall push—for the calves

Stretches

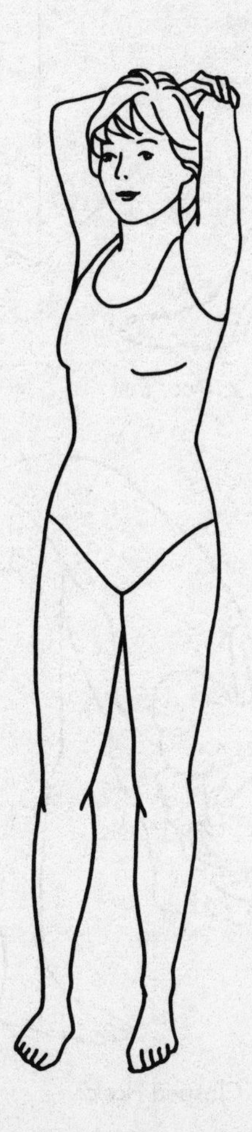

1. Elbow Reach

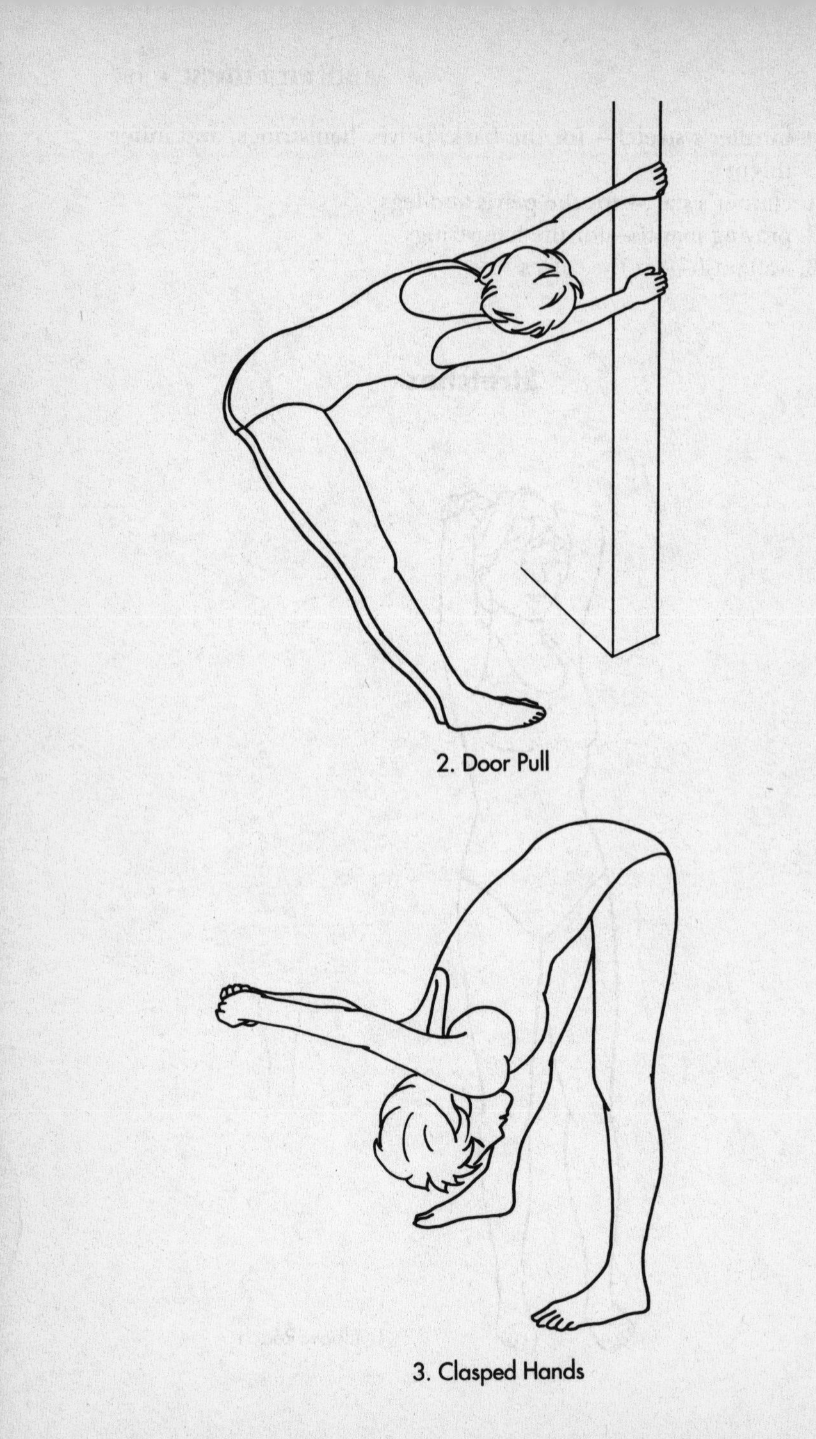

2. Door Pull

3. Clasped Hands

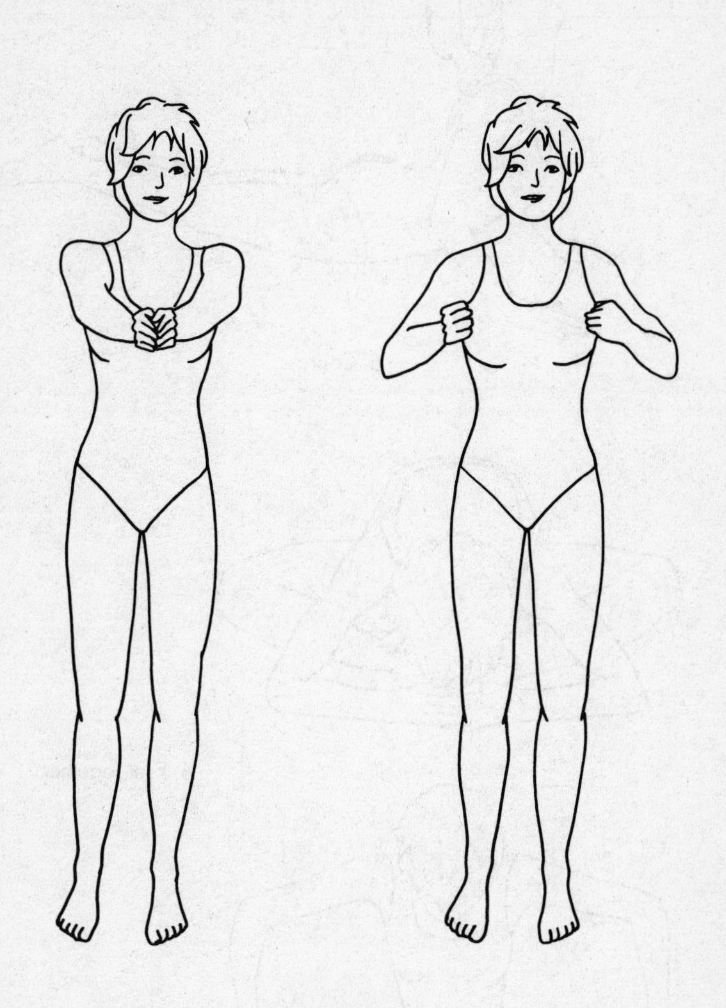

4. Chest Row

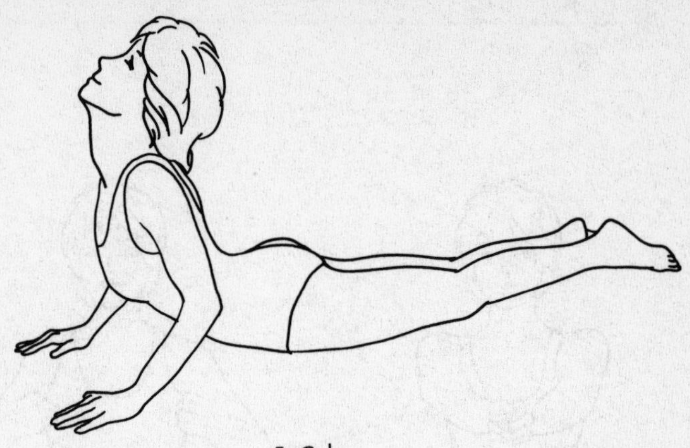

5. Cobra

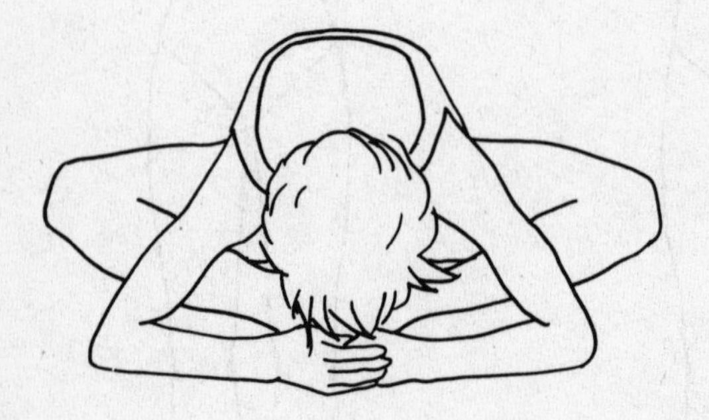

6. Feet Together

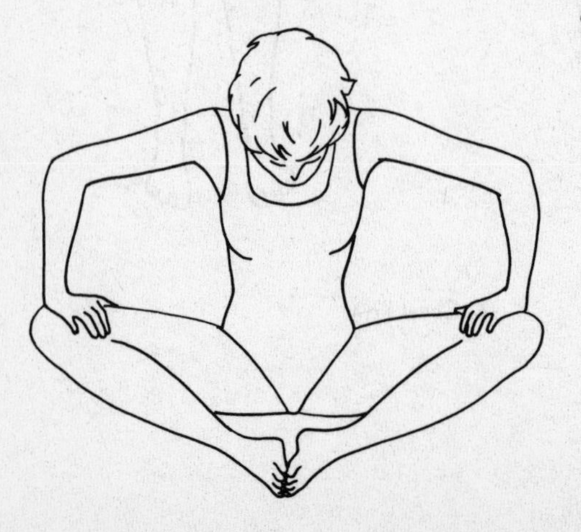

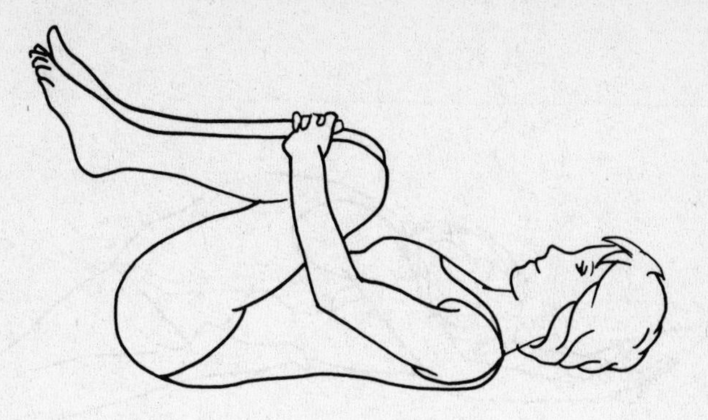

7. Double Knee Hold

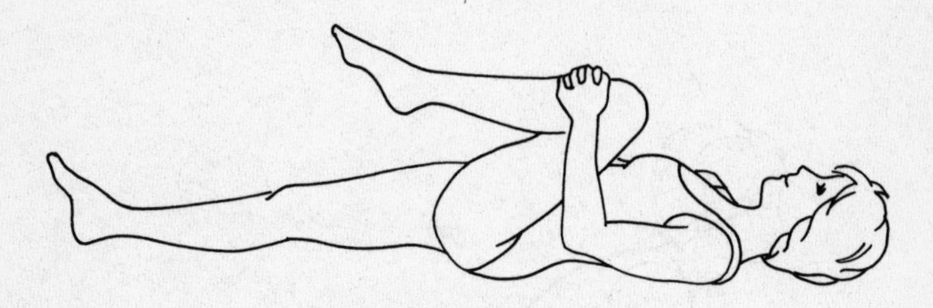

8. One Knee Hold

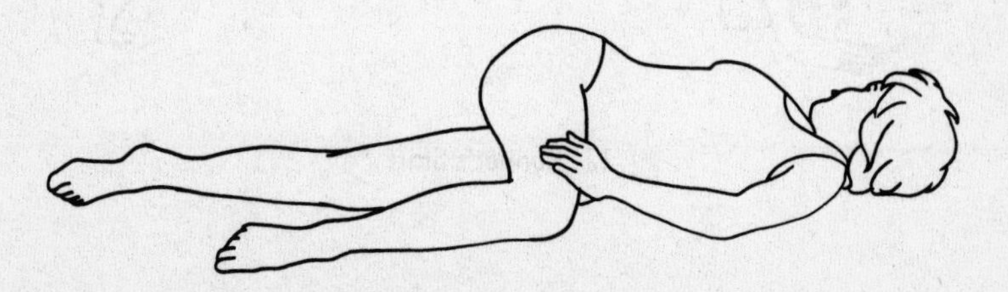

9. Knee Over Trunk

10. Hurdler's Stretch

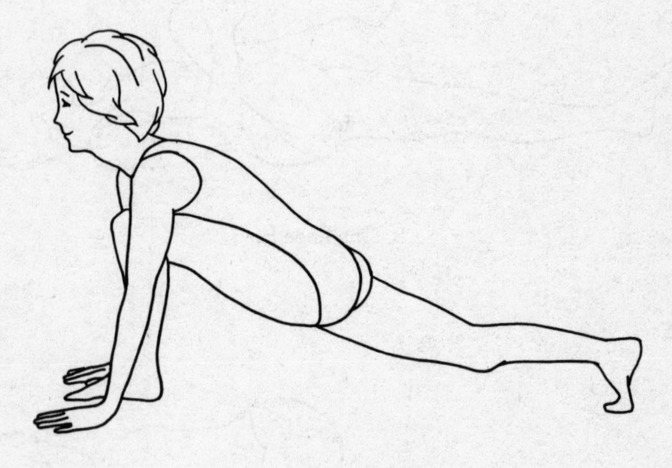

11. Runner's Start

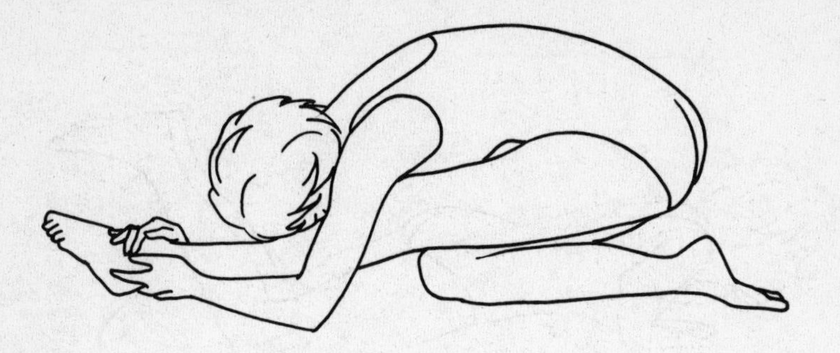

12. Praying Mantis

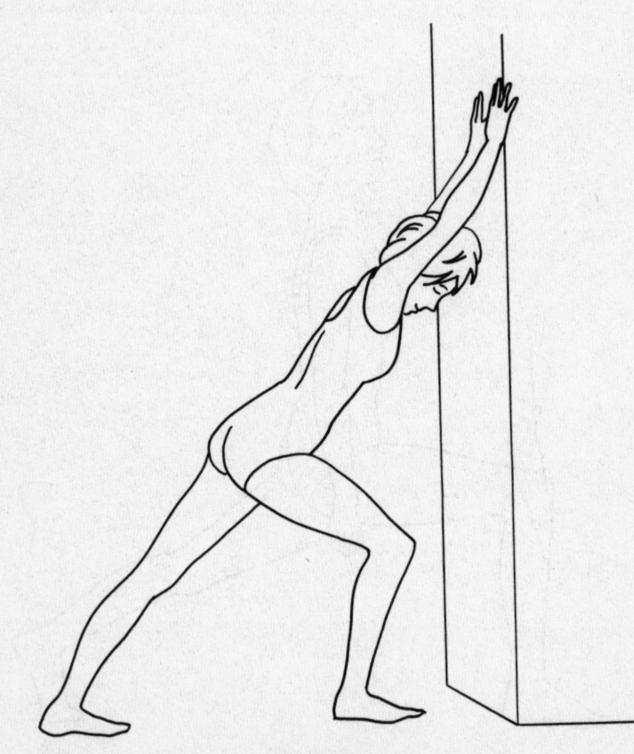

13. Wall Push

Strength-Training Exercises

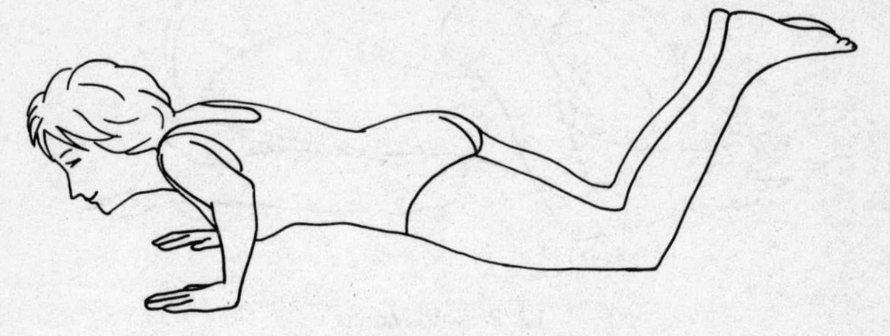

1. Modified Push-Up (no weights)

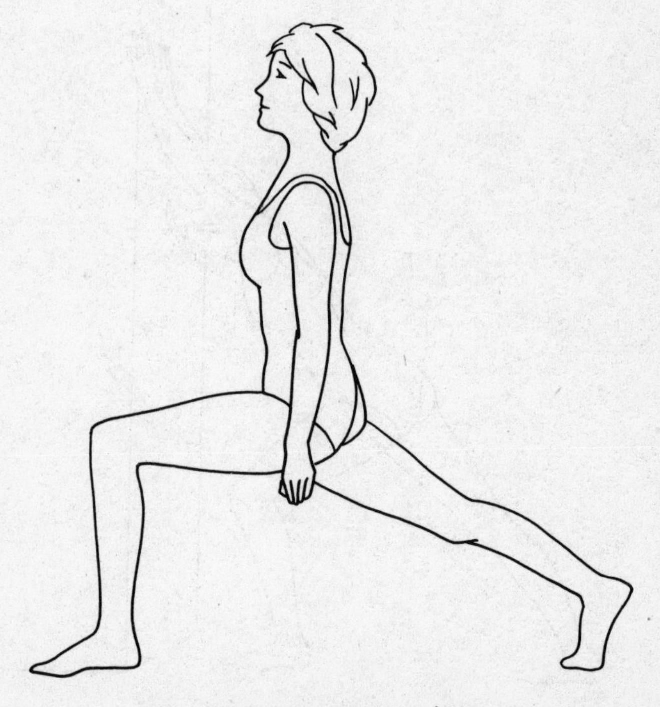

2. Lunges or Stairs (no weights)

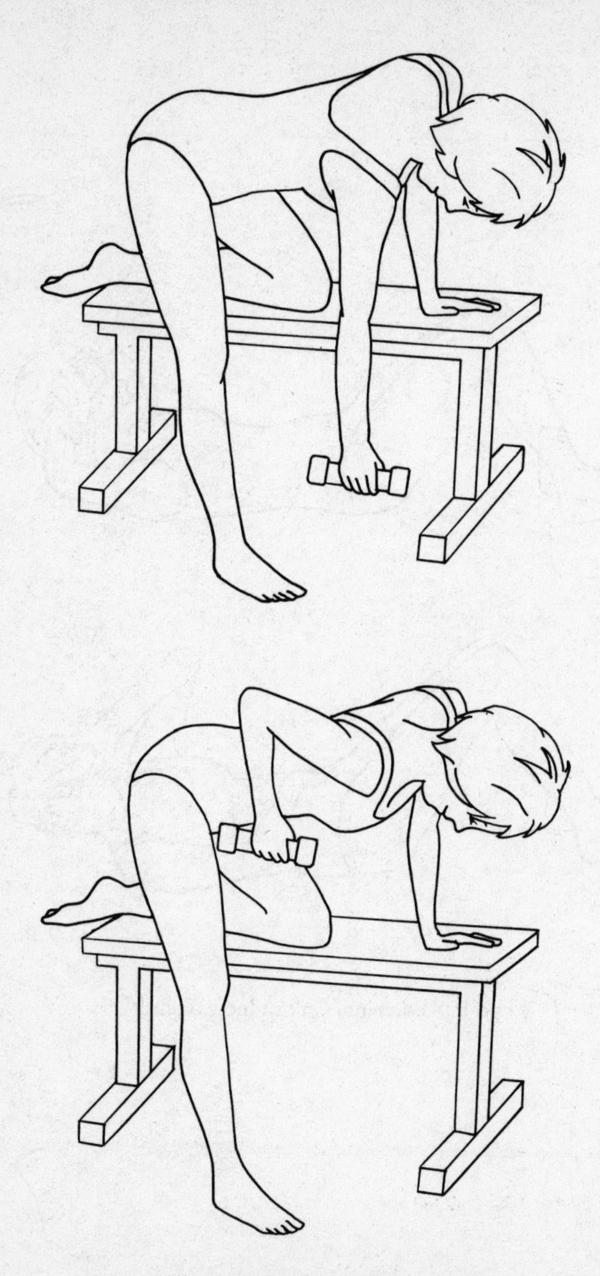

3. Bent Lateral Row (light weights)

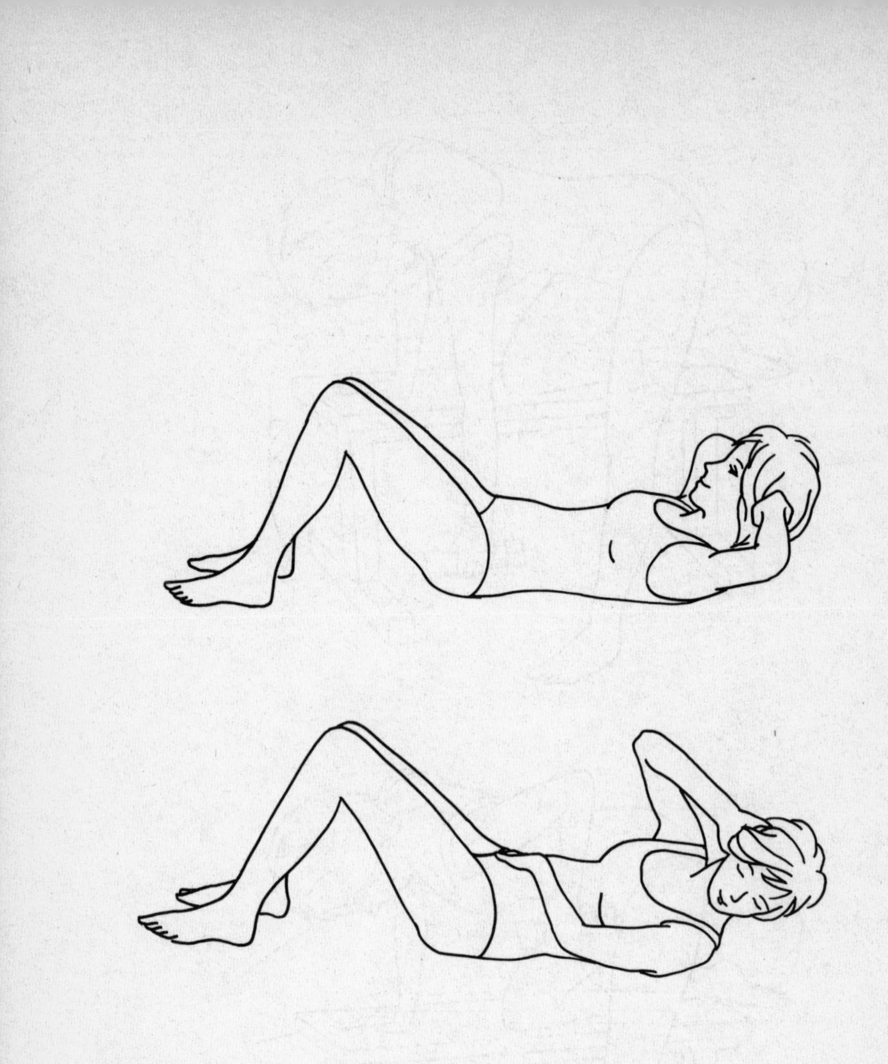

4 and 8. Abdominal Crunch (no weights)

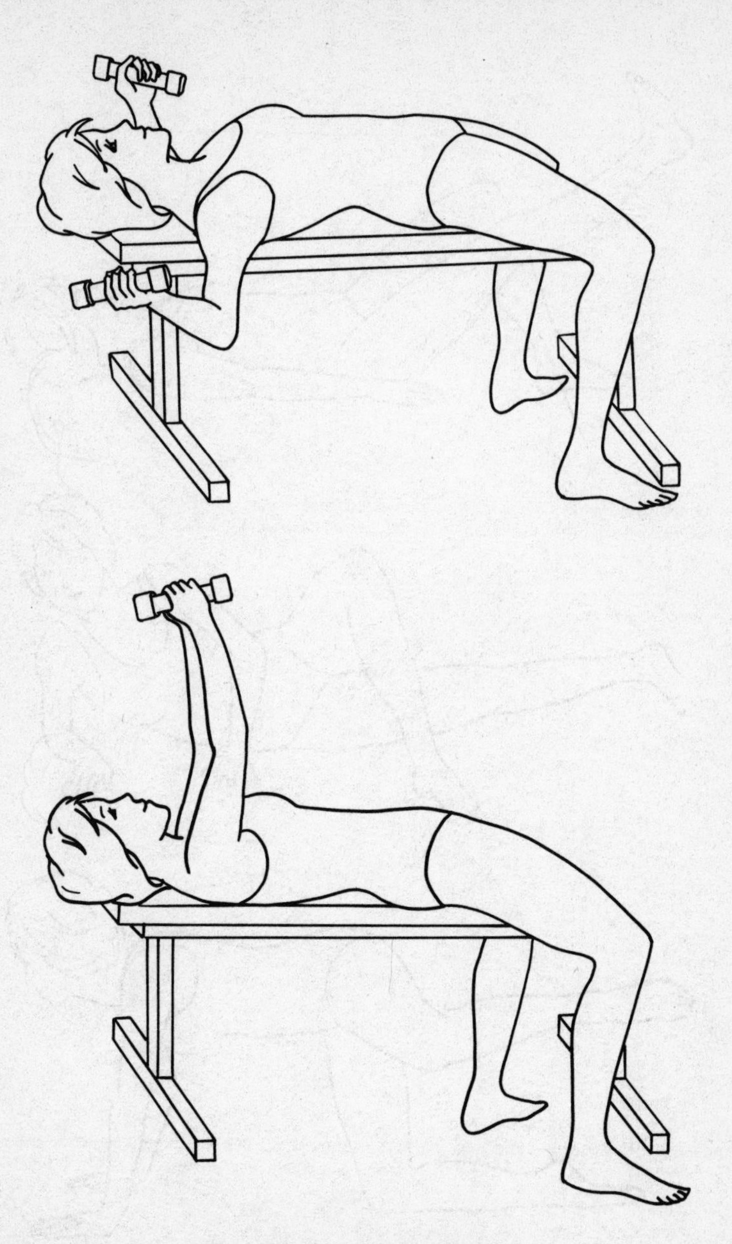

5. Pectoral Fly (medium weights)

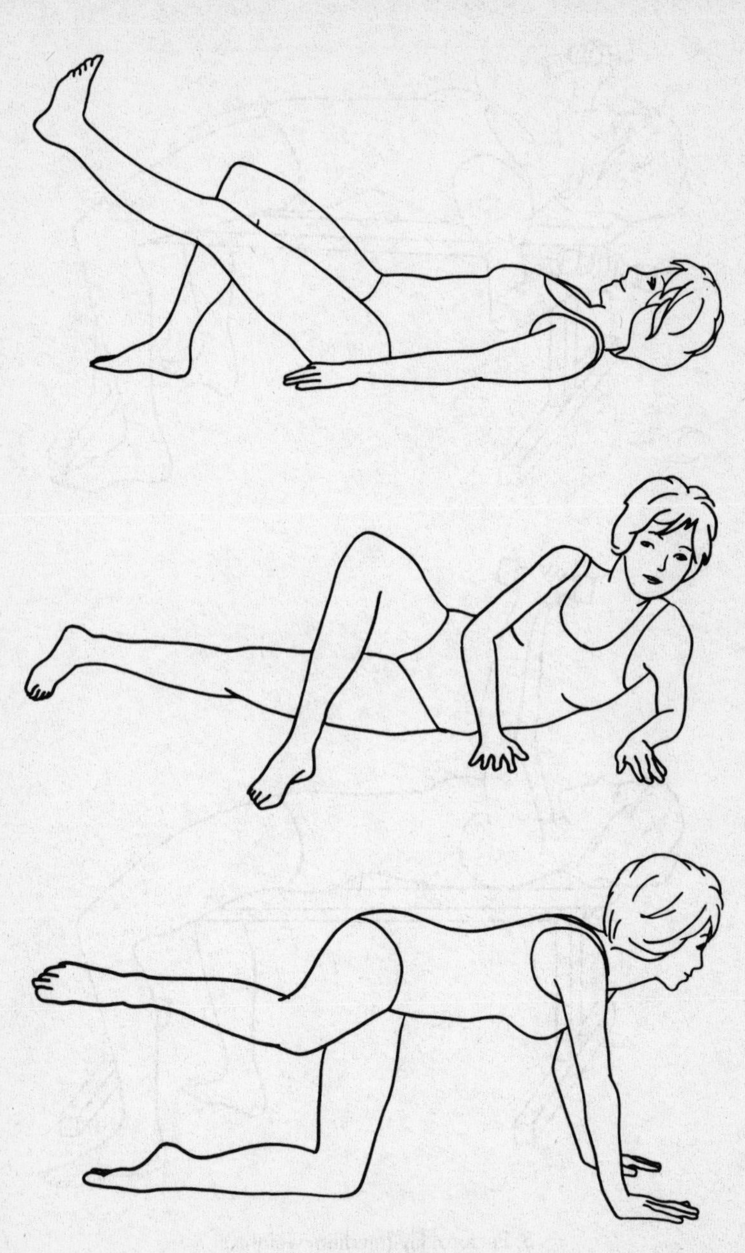

6. Leg Lift

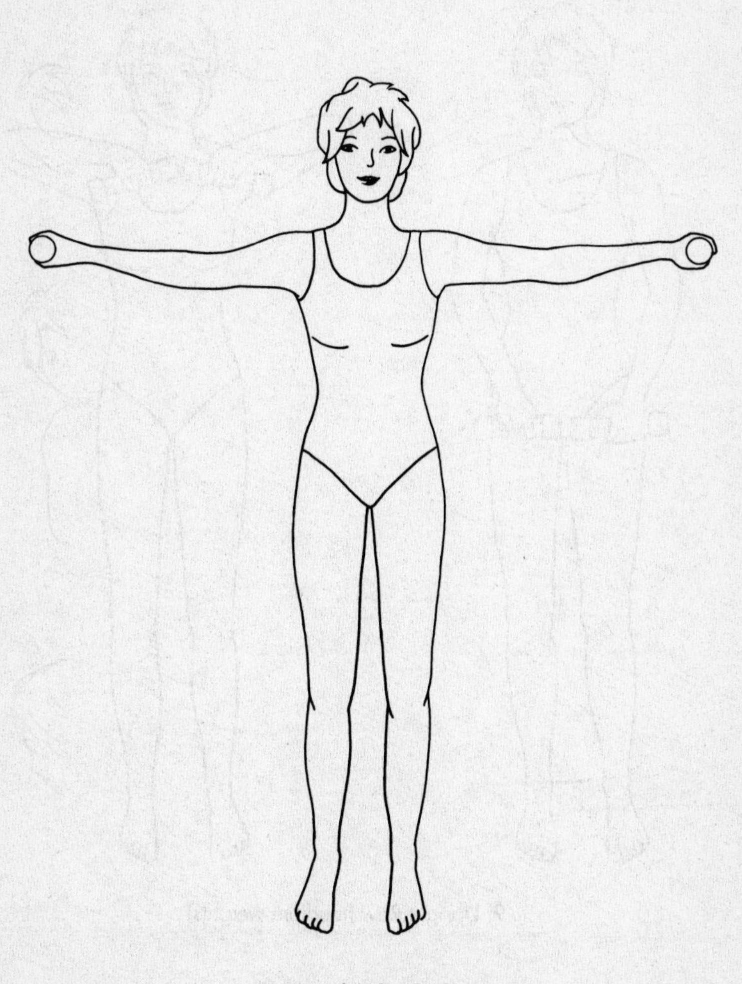

7. Lateral Deltoid Lift

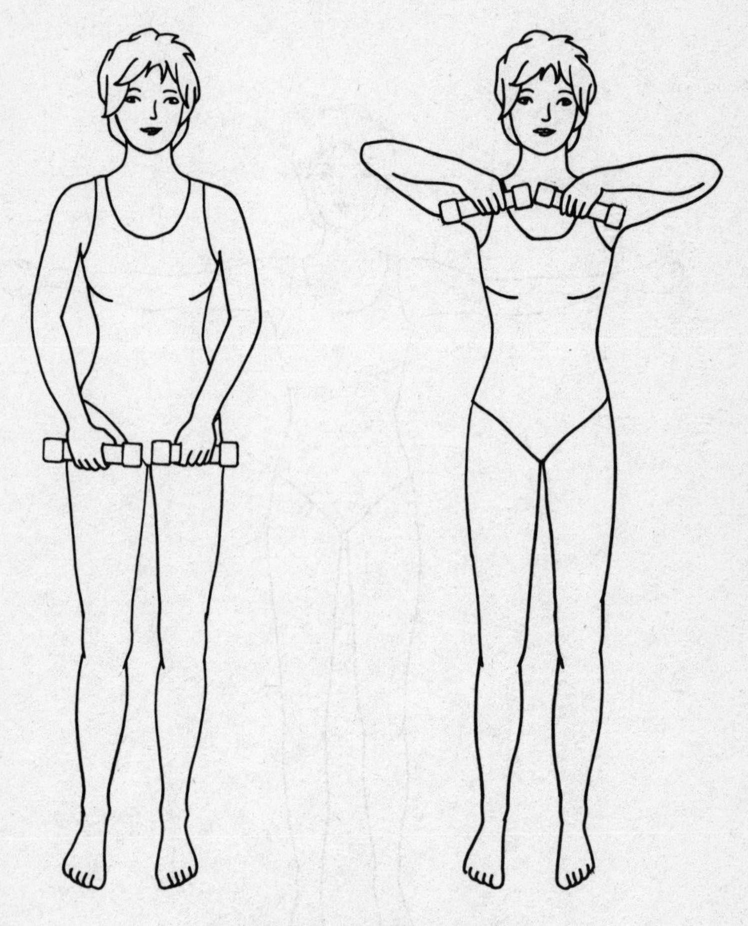

9. Upright Row (medium weights)

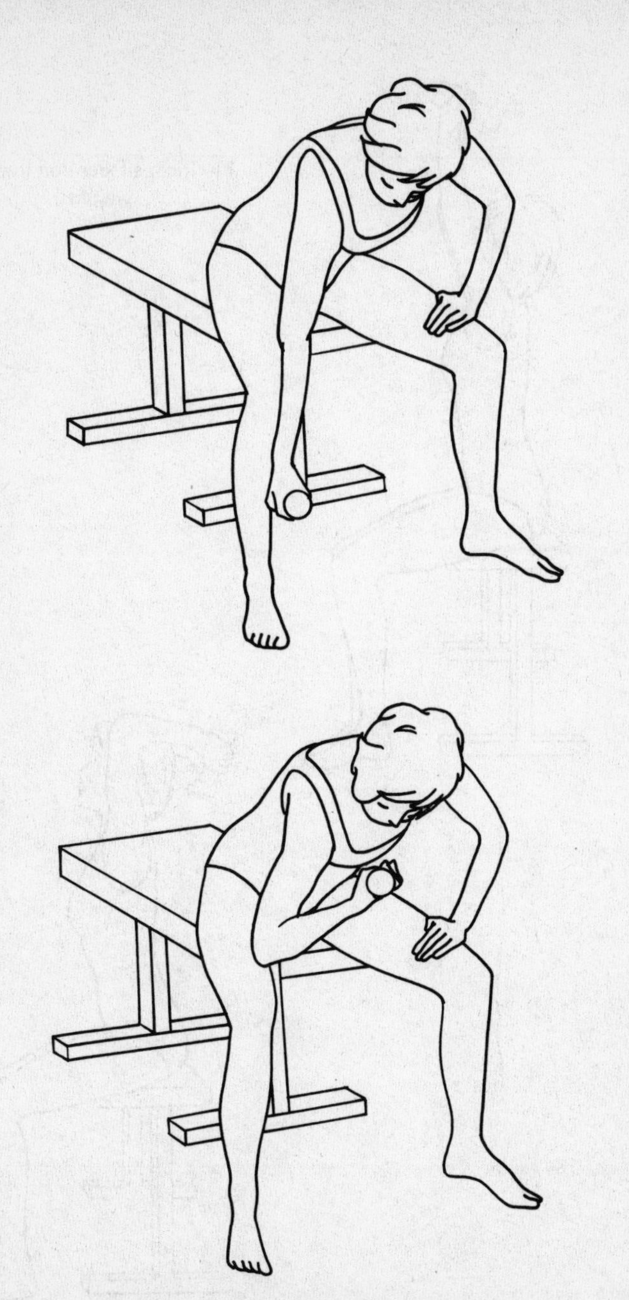

10. Biceps Curl (medium to heavy weights)

11. Triceps Extension (medium weights)

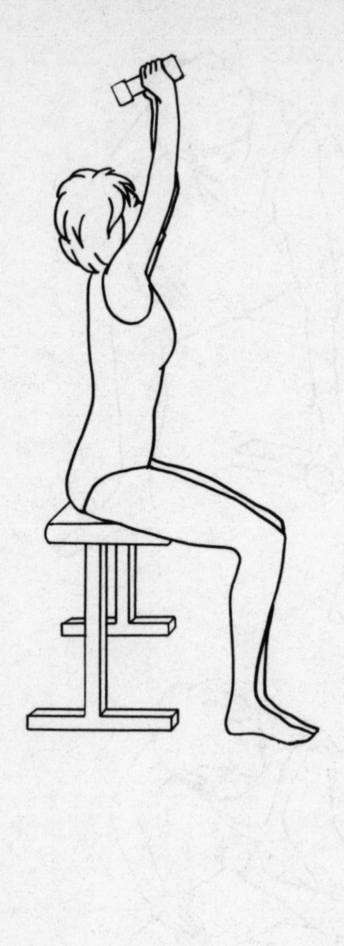

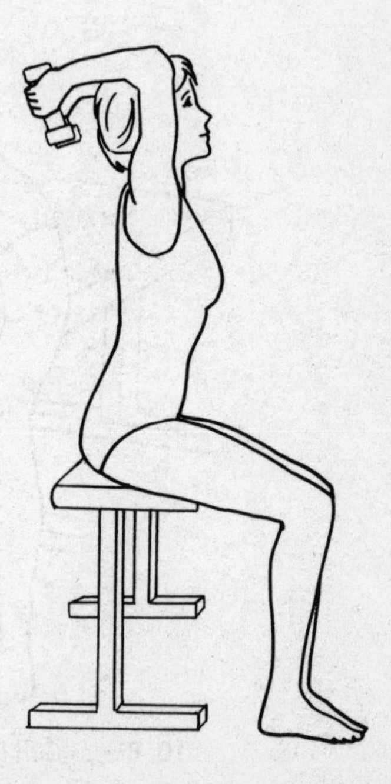

16

A WAY OF LIFE

"It all comes together . . ."

So you will hear over and over from women in their fifties and onward: Life experience combines with new energy, which leads to a feeling of being unshackled from unnecessary restraints and finally living and thinking for oneself. Much has been made in writings about women at midlife of this feeling of *post-menopausal zest,* a phrase coined by Margaret Mead, who discovered in her fifties a renewed vigor, productivity, and love of life. The phenomenon has been attributed to the fact that after menstruation ends, a woman's testosterone-to-estrogen ratio rises, leading to a sense of accelerated well-being and renewed energy. Whatever the specific chemistry behind it, the phenomenon is very real.

Many women experience a profound spiritual awakening at midlife, finding new purpose to their lives—following what the Hindus call *dharma*—and establishing a direct personal connection with the cosmos, or the divine, or however they choose to define it. Some women begin to reconnect in spirit with the ancient goddesses, many of whom in past cultures represented healing with plants—e.g., the Roman goddess Demeter, who represented the harvest, and the Sumerian goddess Gula, who represented healing.

Whatever your personal spiritual inclination, we certainly hope that after reading *Natural Woman, Natural Menopause* you will at least gain a new respect for the *interconnectedness* of all life—that you will come to appreciate the fact that the food you put in your body at lunch, and what comes at you from the environment during the day, can be directly related to that hot flash you have at night.

What can also be awakened at midlife is a more reverential approach to the body, a respect for its own healing powers, and a respect for the traditional healing link to plants for women. Respecting your own body inevitably leads to a sense of revering the planet as well—of doing what you can to keep both it and you healthy at the same time. We cannot be healthy in an unhealthy environment.

Unfortunately, we often only realize how interconnected all life on the planet is when something goes wrong in the ecology—when we start, for example, getting diseases from xenoestrogens. Now more than ever, we can't take good living or good health on this planet for granted.

So look at everything around you in your life. Look to your body. Sometimes we are inclined to treat our bodies as if alien to ourselves and just give them over to others for treatment without question. Take control. Ask questions. Turn "The Change" into an opportunity to more completely understand your body and how you can protect, support, and enhance your hormonal life.

Of primary importance to remember is the avoidance of foreign substances that don't exist in nature. Chemicals that weren't around before man began manipulating nature to profit from it should be approached with great caution. Then examine all your activities, what you eat, what you buy for the household, how you exercise, and do what you can to *clean* it up in every way.

A Kinder, Gentler Medicine

Much of the Western tradition of medicine operates from an "attack" position: It goes to war on disease, uses "antibiotics," and "cuts out the cancers." This attack approach can work for certain conditions—as intervention in emergency medicine it really shines—but it is antithetical to promoting balance and hormonal harmony for women. And the attack approach does inevitably lead to such practices as the unnecessary removal of the uterus, and excessive surgical procedures for everything from bleeding of unknown origin to uterine fibroids, ovarian cysts, cervical dysplasia, and breast lumps. Ultimately, unnecessary surgical interventions set the body up for many other problems, such as increased exposure to anesthetics and antibiotics, all of which can compromise your immune system and create internal imbalance. There is also an increased risk of infections, especially the drug-resistant infections so common in the hospital environment, in addition to surgical adhesions, which then often get treated by further intervention. When you factor all this into taking HRT drugs that don't conform to your native hormones, before you know it you can be led down a road you never wanted to go down and end up a very sick and old woman indeed.

The previous generations of American women were silent on the subject of what happened to their bodies at midlife. A new generation of women is already breaking the chain of silence, and hopefully, when the millions of baby-boom women apply the full force of their intelligence and power to this neglected subject, it will never again be the same. All women will be healthier and more vital for it. Perhaps a new trend can emerge based on the old oral tradition—the passing on from woman to woman of the healing wisdom of Mother Nature and her pharmacy.

We're hoping for the domino effect here. Just in the two years we've spent writing this book, so much has already changed as far as knowledge of "the naturals." In the first months of writing, it felt as if we would be sending a message out mostly into an information void. But soon we began hearing of women who knew about the "hormones from wild yam," even though their knowledge of how they were used was sparse. Then we began to hear of more and more women looking to know more about "the naturals" and telling us, "*When is the book going to be finished? I need the information now.*"

By sharing the relevant information and scientific research with you we hope to help you make better, safer choices. This can lead to support from doctors, which can lead to more and more doctors and pharmaceutical companies coming on board, which will lead to greater acceptance and understanding in the public at large, and, most important of all, to healthier and more vital women who never again will be expected to accept treatments that put them at risk *unnecessarily*, and cause them to suffer side effects *unnecessarily*. Please do your part. Help put a halt to the dangerous trend of putting all women on HRT drugs, with their side effects and long-term risks of cancer. Tell your friends about the new methods you learned in this book.

Spread the word.

Appendix A

DOCTOR REFERRAL LISTINGS AND SUPPORT ORGANIZATIONS

Natural Woman Institute
Founded by Christine Conrad. Through a program of outreach and education for women and physicians, this organization will support a greater understanding of plant-derived hormones, how a woman's body works at mid-life, and how important hormonal balance is to keeping her healthy, active, and vital. A database of doctor referrals will be updated continuously with the latest information.
Phone: 888-4UWOMAN (888-489-6626); or write: NWI, 8539 Sunset Blvd., Suite 135, Los Angeles, California 90069

National College of Naturopathic Medicine
049 SW Porter Street
Portland, Oregon 97201
Phone: 888-NATMEDX (628-6339)

American College for the Advancement of Medicine
P.O. Box 3427
Laguna Hills, California 92654
Phone: 800-532-3688
They require a SASE and $ .55 postage.

American Association of Naturopathic Physicians
P.O. Box 20386
Seattle, Washington 98102
Phone: 206-298-0125
They charge a $5.00 fee for referrals.

North American Menopause Society
This organization will give you the names of doctors in your area who specialize in menopause, but you will have to ask specifically if they are using "the naturals."
University Hospitals
Department of OB/GYN
2074 Abington Road
Cleveland, Ohio 44106
Phone: 216-844-8748
Fax: 216-844-3348

American Academy of Nurse Practitioners
Capitol Station, LBJ Building
P.O. Box 12846
Austin, Texas 78711

Dr. Tori Hudson's A Woman's Time
A menopause clinic.
2067 NW Lovejoy
Portland, Oregon 97209
Phone: 503-222-2322

Dr. Julian Whitaker's *Health and Healing Newsletter*
Phillips Publishing, Inc.
7811 Montrose Road
Potomac, Maryland 20854
Phone: 800-211-8561

Christiane Northrup, M.D., *Health Wisdom for Women*
Phillips Publishing, Inc.
7811 Montrose Road
Potomac, Maryland 20854
Phone: 800-211-8561
This newsletter will provide referrals if you subscribe.

HERS (Hysterectomy Educational Resources and Services)
422 Bryn Mawr Avenue
Bala Cynwyd, Pennsylvania 19004
Phone: 610-667-7757

Women's Health America

Founded by Marla Ahlgrimm, R.Ph., Madison Pharmacy.
P.O. Box 9690
Madison, Wisconsin 53715
Phone: 608-833-9102

Transitions for Health

621 SW Alder, Suite 900
Portland, Oregon 97205
Phone: 800-888-6814

Health World

Excellent on-line resource for complementary medicine. Provides free access to Medline.
http://healthy.net

Appendix B

COMPOUNDING PHARMACIES

Before the era of proprietary phamaceuticals, pharmacists regularly compounded prescriptions to order. They would work with doctors and patients to make exacting prescriptions for the greatest efficacy and the least number of side effects.

By the late sixties and seventies, when pharmaceutical drugs from large manufacturers took over the marketplace, compounding fell into disfavor. Proprietary drugs were originally touted as time-savers, more convenient for pharmacist, doctor, and patient, and capable of generating more profit. Unfortunately, pharmacists increasingly began to be merely purveyors of prefabricated drugs, spending their time counting out pills and filling bottles. These non-compounding pharmacists can provide invaluable services, but not the full range of custom-made natural products available for women's hormonal health.

While researching this book, we were heartened to see that over the last decade, the number of compounding pharmacies and pharmacists is on the upswing, not in small measure due to growing interest in natural plant hormone preparations.

There are a group of pharmacies—Women's International, Madison, Bajamar, Apothecure, Belmar, and College—that specialize in "the naturals" and have very large mail-order businesses. They will send you information packets on "the naturals," plus many of them will provide lists of doctors in your area who use "the naturals" by prescription.

We include here a list of pharmacies that we know compound "the naturals." It is by no means complete, as the number of pharmacies beginning to compound these products is growing rapidly.

International Academy of Compounding Pharmacists
Robert Harshbarger, R.Ph., president; formerly Professionals & Patients for Customized Care; approximately 900 members in the United States, Canada, and Australia. This organization will help you find a compounding pharmacist near you.

P.O. Box 1365
Sugarland, Texas 77487
Phone: 713-933-8400/800-927-4227
Fax: 713-933-9215

The Apothecary

35 Main Street
Keene, New Hampshire 03431
Phone: 603-357-0200
George Roentsch, R.Ph.

Apothecure

Large mail-order business.
13720 Midway Road, Suite 109
Dallas, Texas 75244
Phone: 800-969-6601
Gary Osborn, R.Ph.

Apthorp Pharmacy

2201 Broadway
New York, New York 10024
Phone: 212-877-3480
Tom Giacalone, R.Ph.
Russell Gellis, R.Ph., Owner

Artesia Pharmacy

18550 South Pioneer Boulevard
Artesia, California 90701
Phone: 800-851-7900
Ron Miller, R.Ph.

Bajamar Women's Health Care

Large mail-order business.
9609 Dielman Rock Island
St. Louis, Missouri 63132
Phone: 800-255-8025
Barry Mizes, R.Ph.

Bellgrove Pharmacy

1535 116th Avenue NE
Bellevue, Washington 98004
Phone: 800-446-2123
Mark Holzener, R.Ph.

Belmar Pharmacy

Large mail-order business.
8015 W. Alameda Avenue, Suite 100
Lakewood, Colorado 80226
Phone: 800-525-9473
Charles Hakala, R.Ph.

Birds Hill Pharmacy
401 Great Plains Avenue
Needham, Massachusetts 02192
Phone: 781-449-0550
Hank Abbott, Rosalie Virusso, R.Phs.

California Pharmacy & Compounding Center
307 Placentia Avenue
Newport Beach, California 92663
Phone: 800-575-7776
Steve Feldman, R.Ph.

Cap Rock Pharmacy
2625 50th Street
Lubbock, Texas 79413
David Webb, R. Ph.

College Pharmacy
Large mail-order business.
833 North Tejon Street
Colorado Springs, Colorado 80903
Phone: 800-888-9358
Tom Bader, R.Ph.

Columbine Drugs
2295 W. Eisenhower Boulevard
Loveland, Colorado 80538
Phone: 970-663-7100
Fax: 970-663-7478
Fred Bruno, R.Ph.

Community Pharmacy
117 North Imperial Avenue
Imperial California, 92251
Phone: 760-355-2863
Fax: 760-355-2537
Noel Carrico, R.Ph.

Compounding Pharmacy of Beverly Hills
433 North Roxbury
Beverly Hills, California 90210
Phone: 310-284-8675
Melvin Gross, R.Ph.

Concord Drugs
5555 Peachtree Dunwoody Road, N.E.
Atlanta, Georgia 30342
Phone: 404-252-3607
Mac McCord, R.Ph.

Delk Pharmacy
1602 Hatcher Lane
Columbia, Tennessee 38401
Phone: 616-388-3952
Joe Delk, R.Ph.

Diplomat Pharmacy
3426 Flushing Road
Flint, Michigan 48504
Phone: 810-732-8720
Phil Hagerman, R.Ph.

Doc's Pharmacy
112 La Casa Via, Suite 100
Walnut Creek, California 94598
Phone: 510-939-6311
Robert Horwitz, R.Ph.

Eddie's Pharmacy
8500 Melrose Avenue
West Hollywood, California 90069
Phone: 310-358-2400
Eddie Bubar, R.Ph.

Family Pharmacy
3644 Webber Street
Sarasota, Florida 34232
Phone: 941-921-6645
Fax: 941-923-7758
Mike Pass, R.Ph.

Greenpark Pharmacy
7515 South Main
Houston, Texas 77030
Phone: 713-795-5812
Ken Hughes, R.Ph.

Hospital Discount Pharmacy
104 South Bryant
Edmonds, Oklahoma 73034
Phone: 405-348-1677
Dave Mason, R.Ph.

Jaye Pharmacy
13322 Riverside Drive
Sherman Oaks, California 91423
Phone: 818-789-8111
Reuben Kohan, David Kohan, R.Phs.

Madison Pharmacy Associates
Large mail-order business.
429 Gammon Place
P.O. Box 9641
Madison, Wisconsin 53715
Phone: 800-558-7046
Marla Ahlgrimm, R.Ph.

The Medicine Shoppe
1567 North Eastman Road
Kingsport, Tennessee
Phone: 423-245-1022
Robert Harshbarger, R.Ph.

Mountain View Pharmacy
10565 North Tatum Boulevard, Suite B118
Paradise Valley, Arizona 85253
Phone: 602-948-7065
Evelyn Timmons, R.Ph.

Panorama Pharmacy
8215 Van Nuys Boulevard
Panorama City, California 91402
Phone: 818-988-7979
Fax: 818-787-7256
Earl Broidy, Elaine Blieden, R.Phs.

Phoenix Pharmacy
2523 East Washington Boulevard
Pasadena, California 91104
Phone: 818-791-7600
Jim Avedikian, R.Ph.

PRN Compounders
3030 Burlew Boulevard
Owensboro, Kentucky 42303
Phone: 800-682-5398
Fax: 502-685-5742
David Nation, R.Ph.

Professional Arts Pharmacy
1101 North Rolling Road
Baltimore, Maryland 21225
Phone: 800-832-9285
Sam Georgio, R.Ph.

Rediger's Pharmacy
724 South Eddy, Box 1760
Pecos, Texas 79772
Phone: 800-588-1096
John Rediger, R.Ph.

Shire's Pharmacy
7901 Saltsburg Road
Pittsburgh, Pennsylvania 15239
Phone: 412-792-5230
John Yakim, R.Ph.

South Desert Pharmacy
2600 East Southern Avenue
Tempe, Arizona 85282
Phone: 602-839-0892
Ava Weeks, R.Ph.

Trumarx Drugs
501 Gordon Avenue
Thomasville, Georgia 31792
Phone: 800-552-9997
Marx Gaines, R.Ph.

Universal Arts Pharmacy
6500 W. 4th Avenue, Suite 4
Hialeah/Miami Lakes, Florida 33012
Phone: 305-556-2673
Fax: 305-556-9749
Ray Morano, R.Ph.

University Pharmacy
1320 East 2nd South
Salt Lake City, Utah 84101
Phone: 801-582-7624
Richard Rasmussen, R.Ph.

Wedgewood Village Pharmacy
373 K Egg Harbor Road
Sewell, New Jersey 08080
Phone: 609-589-4200
George Malmberg, R.Ph.

Wellness Health & Pharmaceuticals
2800 South 18th Street
Birmingham, Alabama 35209
Phone: 800-227-2627
Rod Harbin, R.Ph.

Women's International Pharmacy
Large mail-order business. Also in Scottsdale, Arizona.
5708 Monona Drive
Madison, Wisconsin 53716–3152
Phone: 800-279-5708
Wallace Simons, R.Ph.

Appendix C

TESTING AND HORMONE PRODUCT RESOURCES

Aeron Life Cycles Laboratories
1933 Davis Street, Suite 31
San Leandro, California 94557
Phone: 800-631-7900
Fax: 510-729-0383
(specializing in saliva tests for both hormone and bone assays)

Great Smokies Diagnostic Laboratory
18a Regent Park Boulevard
Asheville, North Carolina 28806
Phone: 704-253-0621
Fax: 704-253-1127
E-mail: cs@gsdl.com

Meridien Valley Clinical Laboratory
For steroid hormone profiles.
24030 132nd Avenue SE
Kent, Washington 98042
Phone: 800-234-6285

Metamatrix Medical Research Laboratory
Norcross, Georgia
Phone: 800-221-4640
(Leader in tests for digestive functions and bone assays)

Product Resources

Transitions for Health, Inc. (Pro-Gest®)
621 SW Alder, Suite 900
Portland, Oregon 97205
Phone: 503-226-1010
Phone: 800-888-6814
Enzymatic Therapy: 800-783-2286
Vitanica: 800-572-4712
Prevail: 800-248-0885
Naturally Vitamins: 800-899-4499
Tyler Encapsulatories: 800-869-6705 (doctors only)
Omega Nutrition: 800-661-3529
Phytopharmica: 800-553-2370 (doctors only)
Rx Vitamins: 800-792-2222

Progesterone Content of Body Creams

Aeron LifeCycles has screened a number of commercial cream products with potential hormonal activity for progesterone content as part of an interest in the hormonal activity of natural products and an interest in transdermal hormone supplementation.

Creams Containing More Than 400 Milligrams Progesterone per Ounce of Cream

Pro-Gest	Professional and Technical Services	Portland, OR
Bio Balance	Elan Vitale	Scottsdale, AZ
Progonol	Bezwecken	Beaverton, OR
Ostaderm	Bezwecken	Beaverton, OR
Pro-Alo	HealthWatchers Sys.	Scottsdale, AZ
PhytoGest	Karuna Corp.	Novato, CA
NatraGest	Broadmoore Labs, Inc.	Ventura, CA
Happy PMS	HM Enterprises, Inc.	Norcross, GA
Equilibrium	Equilibrium Lab	Boca Raton, FL
Pro-G	TriMedica	Scottsdale, AZ
ProBalance	Springboard	Monterey, CA

The products listed below do not significantly affect progesterone levels.

Creams Containing 2 to 15 Milligrams Progesterone per Ounce of Cream

Pro-Dermex	Gero Vita International	Reno, NV
Endocreme	Wuliton Labs	Palmyra, MO
Life Changes	MW Labs	Atlanta, GA
Progestone-Plus	Professional Health Products	Sewickley, PA
Novagest	Strata Dermatologics	Concord, CA

Creams Containing Less Than 2 Milligrams or No Progesterone per Ounce of Cream

Yamcon	Phillips Nutritionals	Laguna Hills, CA
Born Again	Phytopharmica	Green Bay, WI
PMS Formula	PMS Relief, Inc.	Auburn, CA
Menopause Form	PMS Relief, Inc.	Auburn, CA
Femarone	Wise Essen, Inc.	Minneapolis, MN
Nutri-Gest	NutriSupplies, Inc.	W. Palm Beach, FL
Progerone	Nature's Nutrition, Inc.	Vero Beach, FL
Wild Yam Cream	Alvin Last, Inc.	Yonkers, NY
Progestone-HP	Dixie Health, Inc.	Atlanta, GA
Woman Wise	Jason Natural Cosmetics	Culver City, CA

(Source: Prepared by Aeron LifeCycles, November 15, 1995)

Appendix D

TRADITIONAL HERBAL REMEDIES

For those women who would prefer an entirely herbal program at midlife—particularly those who are already oriented in that direction—there are a number of traditional herbal remedies that we can recommend. This list is by no means complete, but represents what we think are very good choices. Two of the remedies, gamma oryzanol (rice bran oil) and vitamin E have come into use more recently. Some of these remedies are already included in the preformulated products we recommend in chapter 13, and they are also an option for you.

Recommended Brands:

The following brand names contain high-quality herbal remedies in a variety of combinations or singly: Enzymatic Therapy, Gaia, Zand, Herb Pharm, Eclectic Institute, Naturally, and Tyler Encapsulations.

Chaste Tree Berry (*Vitex agnus castus*)

Recent scientific analysis of this centuries-old remedy has determined that it works by affecting the ratio of LH and FSH hormones, thus helping to balance estrogen and progesterone in the body. It can be taken separately or in combined preparations. It is considered particularly helpful to women who come to menopause early, through either natural or induced means. Because it is considered slow-acting, evidence of effect will only be evident after a few months of daily use.

Dong Quai (*Angelica sinensis*)

This root has been used by the Chinese for thousands of years for gynecological complaints. It is known to have a marked analgesic effect on the uterus, sometimes relaxing, sometimes contracting, as needed. In addition, it has been shown to lower blood pressure, increase the oxygen consumption of the liver, and reduce water retention.[1] It is most often used in combination with other herbs, and, as with many herbal remedies, results will not be evident immediately and may take two weeks.

Licorice Root (*Glycyrrhiza glabra*)

Licorice has been found to possess activity similar to at least two hormones of the adrenal glands, and helps to support normal adrenal function. At midlife, the adrenal glands work to assist the body's hormonal balance by producing low levels of sex hormones.

Ginseng (*Panax ginseng* [Chinese], *Panax quinquefolium* [American], *Eleutherocuccus senticosus* [Siberian])

As an adaptogen, ginseng has overall tonic effects for the body, and because it contains a rich supply of plant hormones, EFAs, antioxidants, minerals, and glycosides, it can be very effective for menopausal symptoms. Since the benefits are cumulative, you must wait two to three weeks before noticing an effect on menopausal symptoms.

Evening Primrose Oil

This traditional remedy of the North American Indians is frequently used for PMS and menopausal symptoms. It contains GLA, an essential fatty acid that the body does not manufacture and which must be supplied through diet. It has been the subject of numerous recent studies,[2] and is known to help prevent hardening of the arteries, heart disease, PMS, and high blood pressure. It has also been show to be anti-inflammatory and to have a regulating effect on the prostaglandins.

Wild Yam (*Dioscorea villosa*)

The wild yam in its unsynthesized state has been a remedy for "women's complaints" for thousands of years. When used in its natural state, it does not convert to progesterone directly, but has a balancing effect on your native hormones. It has been used traditionally to prevent miscarriage and ease menstrual pain and menopausal symptoms. It is frequently included in combination herbal products for women at midlife.

Gamma Oryzanol

This is an extract from rice bran oil. It is a safe and nontoxic natural food derivative that has been shown in recent studies to be effective for menopausal symptoms. A Japanese study done in 1984 reported the results of women who took 300 milligrams per day of gamma oryzanol. They showed an 85 percent improvement in their menopausal symptoms within two months.[3]

Brands we recommend: Tyler Encapsulations' gamma oryzanol, and Prevail's MENO-FEM. These products contain gamma oryzanol plus other supporting synergists.

Vitamin E

Taken daily, vitamin E has been shown to improve menopausal symptoms such as hot flashes and night sweats. In one study, women who took only 50–100 IUs per day reduced their hot flashes and night sweats by 75 percent in just four weeks.[4] In another study involving doses of vitamin E of as little as 25 IUs daily over two weeks to three months, over half of the women had improvements in hot flashes, sweats, backaches, muscle pains, and heavy bleeding. When the dose was doubled or quadrupled, over 75 percent of this study group had improvement in hot flashes and sweats, over 85 percent had relief from backaches, joint aches, and headaches, 70 percent of the patients had relief from fatigue, and nearly that many had relief from nervousness.

Vitamin E can have very important benefits for women in the prevention of heart diseases. The Nurses' Health Study used data from 87,245 women, ages 34 to 59, who were free of heart disease in 1980. After adjusting for age, smoking, obesity, exercise, and other risk factors, researchers found that nurses who took vitamin E supplements had only two thirds the risk for heart attack compared to those not taking supplements. Women taking vitamin E for more than two years had only about half the risk.

When we refer to vitamin E we mean natural vitamin E, d-alpha tocopherol, or perhaps d-alpha plus mixed tocopherols. You can buy this in an oil base or in a dry form. If you buy one of our recommended brands, the oil is less expensive and is preferred. We strongly recommend that you take supplemental vitamin E only if you are supplementing with your multivitamin and mineral and antioxidant doses, at the least. If you take it by itself, it won't be as effective.

Brands we recommend: Grace Unique Vitamin E, Naturally's Mixed E 400, Kal Vitamin E 400.

Take 100 to 800 IUs daily, in divided doses, with meals.

Appendix E

RECOMMENDED ORGANIC PRODUCTS AND RESOURCES

The health food industry is constantly growing and changing. Please consider this list a partial resource and continue to do your own research into new companies. More important, we encourage you to support your community natural food stores, delis, restaurants, organic farmers, and local health-supportive cooks. Many of the national natural food store chains like Whole Foods Market and Wild Oats now make many private label organic products. Remember to read your labels.

Cookies: Barbara's, Westbrae, Heaven Scent
Crackers: Barbara's, Health Valley, Edward and Sons, Hain
Tomato sauce: Glen Muir, Millina's Finest, Eden, Garden Valley, and Evy's Garden
Pasta: Eden, Millina's Finest, Mendocino Pasta Company, Westbrae
To-go soups: Nile Spice, Fantastic Foods
Beans: Arrowhead Mills, Eden, Bearitos, Westbrae
Cereals: Nature's Path, Barbara's, Health Valley, Erewhon, and Arrowhead Mills
Grains and flours: Arrowhead Mills, Lundberg
Juices: Santa Cruz, R.W. Knudsen, Mountain Sun
Sparkling fruit drinks (spritzers): R.W. Knudsen, Crystal Geyser
Milk and dairy products (milk, yogurt, cheese, butter, etc.): Horizon, Alta Dena, and Strauss Family

Milk (soy, rice, and almond): Eden, Westbrae, Rice Dream, Wholesome & Hearty
Amasake and mochi: Grainaissance
Teas: Choice, Stash, Eden, Celestial Seasoning
Tamari: San-J, Oshawa, Eden
Miso: Miso Master
Tofu: Nasoya
Mustard and catsup: Westbrae, Garden Valley
Soy cheese: Soya Kaas, Vegan Rella
Jams and jellies: Cascadian Farms, R.W. Knudsen, Sorrel Ridge
Nut butters: Arrowhead Mills, Maranatha
Chips, popcorn, and pretzels: Kettle Chips, Mexi-Snax, Barbara's, Bearitos, Garden of Eatin', Westbrae and Newman's Own
Salad dressings: Spectrum Naturals, Annies, Paula's, Simply Delicious, Nasoya, Ayla's, Paul Newman's
Oils: Omega Nutrition, Barleen's, Spectrum Naturals, Arrowhead Mills
Frozen foods: Cascadian Farms, Amy's, Imagine Foods, Wholesome & Hearty
Ice Cream: Cascadian Farms, Stoneyfield, Imagine Foods, Rice Dream

Another great resource for organics: The *1996 National Organic Directory* lists organic farmers, wholesalers, and businesses by region, and includes a marketing guide and index of more than 1,000 organic commodities. Their phone number is 800-852-3832.

Appendix F

RECOMMENDED COOKBOOKS

There are many excellent cookbooks you can find that feature recipes for applying the Natural Woman eating plan. We list below a cross section of some of the most recent and notable.

Dean Ornish, M.D., *Everyday Cooking with Dr. Dean Ornish* (New York: HarperCollins, 1996).

Earl Mindell, R.Ph., Phd., *Earl Mindell's Soy Miracle* (New York: Simon & Schuster, 1995).

Ruth Winter, *Super Soy, The Miracle Bean* (New York: Crown, 1996).

Bessie Jo Tillman, M.D., *The Natural Healing Cookbook* (Rudra Press, 1995).

Jane Fonda, *Cooking for Healthy Living* (Turner Publishing, 1996).

Bob Greene and Oprah Winfrey, *Make the Connection* (New York: Hyperion, 1996).

Julee Rosso, *Fresh Start* (New York: Crown, 1996).

Nina Shandler, *Estrogen, the Natural Way* (New York: Villard, 1997).

Appendix G

LIST OF MENOPAUSAL SYMPTOMS

hot flashes
night sweats
vaginal dryness
vaginal odor
vaginal atrophy
mood swings
irritability
insomnia
depression
hair growth on face
painful sex
loss of sexual desire
urinary tract infections
weird dreams
lower back pain
itching of the vulva
bloatedness
flatulence
indigestion
osteoporosis
aching ankles, knees, wrists, shoulders
sore heels
thinning scalp
frequent urination
snoring
sore breasts
palpitations
urinary leakage
swollen veins
dizzy spells
vertigo
panic attacks
migraine headaches
skin feeling crawly
memory lapses

GLOSSARY

adaptogen — a safe herbal substance that helps the body cope with stress, tension, anxiety, or physical strain. Adaptogens have a balancing effect on the body.

adrenal glands — two glands about the size of a thumb located on top of the kidneys, which secrete steroid hormones—including cortisol, aldosterone, DHEA, and the stress hormones epinephrine and norepinephrine. The body's shock absorbers, they determine the body's response to stress.

amenorrhea — the absence of menstrual bleeding in a woman who is premenopausal, the cause of which can be varied.

amino acids — the building blocks of protein molecules, necessary for every bodily function. There are twenty different types of amino acids, which come in two forms: *nonessential,* which the body can produce for itself, and *essential,* which the body must extract from food.

androgenic — produces masculine changes in the body. Androgenic substances can be either natural or synthetic and the changes can be male-pattern hair growth, oily skin, acne, deepening of the voice, increased appetite, increased muscle mass, and increased total cholesterol with lower HDL.

androgens — hormones, e.g., testosterone, DHEA, androstenedione, produced by the adrenal glands and gonads (ovaries in the woman, testes in the man) that promote masculine changes in the body. Androgens are produced in smaller amounts in women, but in the postmenopausal woman they go up, thus explaining the characteristic changes seen in older women.

anovulatory — lack of ovulation.

antibody — protein produced in the body to bind with antigens and help neutralize, inhibit, or destroy them.

antigen — a substance that causes an immune system reaction with an antibody. Bacteria, viruses, pollen, dust, mold, and incompletely digested food are common antigens.

antioxidant — a chemical compound that neutralizes the cell-damaging free radicals that are created when oxygen is utilized inside the body's cells. In combating free radicals, antioxidants appear to protect against cancer and possibly other diseases. The principal antioxidant nutrients are: beta-carotene, vitamins C and E, and the mineral selenium. Free radicals are atoms or groups of atoms that can cause damage to our cells, impairing our immune systems and leading to infections and various degenerative diseases.

atherosclerosis — when fatty substances (cholesterol and triglycerides) are deposited in the arteries; this can eventually lead to blockage of the arteries.

carcinogenic — a substance or agent capable of causing cancer.

cholesterol — produced by the liver or obtained through food, this fat-like substance is essential for the production of cell membranes, sex hormones, and vitamin D, among other things. High levels, however, have been associated with an increased risk of developing atherosclerosis and coronary heart disease.

conjugated — in biochemistry, refers to one compound combined with another. Premarin contains "conjugated" estrogens.

corpus luteum — after the release of the egg during ovulation, the yellow-colored, progesterone-producing sac that is formed within the ovary from the remains of the follicle.

daidzein — a powerful isoflavone from soybeans shown to have anticarcinogenic properties.

DHEA — an androgenic hormone produced in the adrenal cortex, gonads, and brain. It is a precursor hormone, meaning that other steroid hormones are made from it. Low levels of DHEA in the blood are a marker for many degenerative diseases.

diosgenin — a substance derived from wild yams that can, in the laboratory, be altered to produce a number of steroids, including pregnenolone (a precursor to DHEA) and progesterone. It does not appear to be possible for the body to make this conversion, but diosgenin may provide other health benefits.

dysmenorrhea — painful menstruation.

endocrine — the hormone-secreting glands.

endogenous — coming from within the body.

endometrium — the mucous membrane lining of the uterus.

enzymes — catalysts (generally proteins) that facilitate or speed up specific chemical reactions.

ERT — estrogen replacement therapy, the most common form of prescription estrogen therapy that uses only estrogen and no progesterone or progestin.

essential fatty acids — fatty acids necessary for cellular metabolism that the body cannot manufacture and that must be obtained through diet. Good sources are fish oils, oils from nuts and seeds, and evening primrose oil.

estradiol (E2) — the most common circulating hormone in premenopausal women.

estriol (E3) — produced in large amounts during pregnancy, it is the "weakest" of the primary human estrogens.

estrogen — a class of hormones important in promoting female characteristics. Men also produce them but in lesser amounts.

estrone (E1) — the most common circulating hormone in postmenopausal women, thought to be one of the culprits in increased risks of endometrial and breast cancers.

follicle — a pod or pouch composed of cells, as in the ovarian follicle, which produces the ovum. When the follicle opens, the egg is discharged and is then picked up by the fallopian tube for transportation into the uterus.

free radicals — highly reactive substances in the body, produced by normal metabolism. They are carefully regulated by other substances and enzymes called free-radical scavengers, or antioxidants. Free radicals are also produced by radiation and industrial pollution. Unfortunately, this extra exposure may inhibit the body's control mechanism and lead to free-radical damage. Free-radical damage is believed to be responsible, at least in part, for a wide range of disorders, including heart disease and cancer.

FSH (follicle stimulating hormone) — involved in a woman's monthly cycle. At the beginning of the cycle, the pituitary gland releases FSH, which stimulates the ovaries to develop and enlarge several follicles, or human egg cells.

genistein — an isoflavone exclusively found in soy that has been shown in studies to inhibit both breast and prostate cancer. It has also been shown to turn cancer cells into normal cells, thus stopping the spread of cancer.

GLA (gamma-linolenic acid) — an omega-6 essential fatty acid that has an antiinflammatory effect in the body. It is used to synthesize prostaglandins.

HDL (high-density lipoprotein) — the body's major carrier of cholesterol to the liver for excretion in the bile. It is called the "good" cholesterol.

hormone — a chemical substance circulating in the body fluids that is a product of living cells and that produces a specific effect on the activity of cells remote from its point of origin. Hormones signal enzymes to perform their function relative to blood sugar levels, insulin levels, menstrual cycles, and growth.

HRT — hormone replacement therapy, or the administration of hormones for the replacement of hormones no longer being produced by the body. The most common form now being prescribed is generally a combination of an estrogenic drug with the addition of progestins.

hypothalamus — a gland found deep in the brain that plays a role in mood, appetite, and the functions of the hormonal and autonomic nervous systems.

isoflavones — compounds found in plant foods such as soy that resemble natural estrogens produced in the body and that are mildly estrogenic. Many of these compounds are believed to protect against cancer.

LDL — low-density lipoprotein, which carries cholesterol through the bloodstream. Sometimes referred to a "bad" cholesterol, studies have shown that high levels can enhance the risk of coronary heart disease.

legume — a plant food group that includes soybeans, peas, lentils, and kidney beans.

lignan — plant fiber reputed to have antiestrogenic activity. The best source of lignan is flaxseed.

LH — the luteinizing hormone, produced by the pituitary gland. When combined with FSH, the two stimulate the ovary to secrete estrogen and begin ovulation. It is also responsible for the development of the corpus luteum. LH levels rise dramatically during menopause and stay elevated throughout post-menopause.

luteal phase — the second half of the menstrual cycle, when progesterone is dominant (from ovulation until menses).

lycopene — an antioxidant found in tomatoes.

lysine — an essential amino acid usually missing from plant foods but found in soybeans.

menopause — the cessation of menstrual cycles.

metabolism — physical and chemical processes that take place in the body to build up and maintain living tissue and to provide energy.

micronize — to reduce a substance to particles only a few microns in diameter.

miso — a fermented paste from soybeans frequently used in soups.

nutraceutical — naturally occurring non-nutritional substance in plants and foods that have physiologic activity but are not classified as a drug.

oophorectomy — the surgical removal of the ovaries.

osteoblast — a bone cell that forms new bone.

osteoclast — a bone cell that resorbs old bone.

pathogen — any agent that causes a disease, especially a microorganism such as a bacterium or fungus.

peri-menopause — the time before menopause when hormonal changes are occurring and periods are starting to be skipped. Peri-menopause can last through the first few years of menopause after periods stop. The age at onset is variable and can be accompanied by cholesterol changes, sleep changes, hot flashes, and bone loss.

phytic acid — a compound found in soy. Studies have shown it to inhibit the growth of tumors in animals.

phyto — denotes a relationship to plants.

phytochemicals — chemicals found in plants that are thought to be protective against disease.

phytoestrogen — a compound structurally similar to human estrogen that is found in plants. It can bind with estrogen receptors in the body and is believed to be protective in breast and prostate cancer, which are both hormone-dependent cancers.

phytohormone — a hormone found in plants.

phytonutrient — a nutrient coming from plants.

phytosterol — a hormone found in plants (used interchangeably with phytohormone).

post-menopause — the years after the cessation of menstruation.

progesterone — a natural ovarian hormone made by the corpus luteum to sustain the endometrium and support the fertilized ovum.

progestin — a synthetic form of progesterone (also known as medroxyprogesterone acetate or megestrol acetate); also known as progestogen, principally in England, and gestogen, in Europe.

prostaglandins — chemicals composed of fatty acids that have a hormonelike effect. They influence muscular contractions, circulation, and inflammation; can regulate cell behavior and inhibit hormones.

resorption — the dissolving away of a substance.

serum — the watery, noncellular liquid of the blood.

sex hormones — the hormones involved in sex determination, function, and characteristics.

steroids — usually refers to hormones with molecular shape similar to cholesterol, i.e., composed of joined rings.

sterol — an organic compound composed of joined rings, making it a fat-soluble alcohol. The most well-known sterol is cholesterol.

tempeh — a fermented soy product with a nutty texture.

testosterone — the major male sex hormone produced in the testes, which also appears in smaller amounts in women (produced by the ovary).

thyroid gland — the endocrine gland in front of the larynx that produces the predominant hormones of metabolism, thyroxine and triiodothyronine.

uterus — the female organ that carries a growing fetus, also known as the womb.

xenobiotics — non-natural substances, almost always petrochemically based, that have a hormonelike effect on the body and can be detrimental to overall hormone balance.

xenoestrogens — a class of xenobiotics that has a specifically estrogenic effect on the body, which can interfere with normal hormone balance.

NOTES

Chapter 1: Another Way

1. "Old Age Elixir?" *Los Angeles Times,* December 13, 1994, pp. E1–E7, reporting on the increase in doctors prescribing hormone replacement therapy.
2. This figure was determined by our survey of compounding pharmacists and producers of over-the-counter products.
3. Panelist Dr. Susan Love at "Women and Doctors," UCLA symposium, May 1994.
4. Gail Sheehy, *The Silent Passage* (New York: Random House, 1991), 56–59.
5. As reported in the *Los Angeles Times,* March 27, 1996, p. E1–2.
6. Germaine Greer, *The Change* (New York: Ballantine, 1991), 144.
7. P. Cotton, "FDA lifts ban on women in early drug test, will require companies to look for gender differents," *Journal of the American Medical Association* 269, no. 16 (1993): 2067(1); also "Testing Drugs in People," *FDA Consumer* 28, no. 6 (July–August 1994): 16(4).
8. Claudia Wallis, "The Estrogen Dilemma," *Time,* June 26, 1995, pp. 46–53.
9. Graham A. Colditz, Susan E. Hankinson, et al., "The use of estrogens and progestins and the risk of breast cancer in postmenopausal women," *New England Journal of Medicine* 332, no. 24 (June 15, 1995): 1589–93.
10. "Old Age Elixir," *Los Angeles Times,* December 13, 1994, pp. E1–7.
11. Sheehy, *The Silent Passage,* 165–74.
12. *Los Angeles Times,* "Natural Selection," November 10, 1995, pp. E1–8.
13. Jerilynn Prior, "Progesterone as a Bonetrophic Hormone," *Endocrine Reviews* 11, no. 2 (May 1990): 387–97.
14. "Progesterone May Play Major Role in the Prevention of Nerve Diseases," *The New York Times,* June 27, 1995, p. C3.
15. King-Jen Chang, et al., "Influences of percutaneous administration

of estradiol and progesterone on human breast epithelial cell cycle in vivo," *Fertility and Sterility* 3, no. 4 (April 1995): 785–791.

16. Elizabeth Vliet, *Screaming to Be Heard* (New York: M. Evans, 1996), 113.
17. Herman Aldercreutz, et al., "Urinary excretion of lignans and isoflavanoid phytoestrogen in Japanese men and women consuming a traditional Japanese diet," *American Journal of Clinical Nutrition* 54 (1991): 1093–1100.
18. R. E. Frisch, et al., "Lower prevalence of breast cancer and cancers of the reproductive system among former college athletes compared to nonathletes," *British Journal of Cancer* 52 (1985): 885–91.
19. Judith K. Brown, et al., *In Her Prime* (South Hadley, Mass.: Bergin & Garvey, 1985), 23–33.

Chapter 2: "Estrogen": The Misunderstood Hormone

1. Egon Diczfalusy, "The Early History of Estriol," *Journal of Steroid Biochemistry* 20, no. 48, 945.
2. Alvin H. Follingstad, "Estriol, the forgotten estrogen?" *Journal of the American Medical Association* 239, no. 1 (January 2, 1978): 29–30.
3. B. Sherwin and L. Kampen, "Estrogen Use and Verbal Memory in Healthy Post-Menopausal Women," *Obstetrics and Gynecology* 83, no. 6 (June 1994): 979–83.
4. Reuters news release, November 5, 1996. Premarin described as "most widely prescribed drug in the U.S."
5. Sheehy, *The Silent Passage,* 207–8.
6. Herman Aldercreutz, et al., "Dietary Phyto-estrogens and the menopause in Japan" (letter) *Lancet* 339 (1992): 1233.
7. Margaret Lock, "Contested meanings of the menopause," *Lancet,* May 25, 1991, referring to K. M. Weiss, "Evolutionary Perspectives on Aging," in *Other Ways of Growing Old,* P. T. Amoss and S. Harrell, eds. (Stanford: Stanford University Press, 1981), 25–28.
8. Jeanne Louise Calment, born February 2, 1875, living in Arles, France.
9. Honora E. Wolfe, *Mènopause: A Second Spring* (Boulder, CO: Blue Poppy Press, 1993), 26–28.

Chapter 3: The Power of Plant Hormones

1. Peter Tompkins and Christopher Bird, *The Secret Life of Plants* (New York: Harper & Row, 1973), viii.
2. Ibid., ix.
3. John Finnegan, *The Facts About Fats* (Malibu, CA: Elysian Arts, 1992), 2.
4. Barbara Griggs, *Green Pharmacy* (Rochester, VT: Healing Arts Press, 1981), 6.
5. Jeanne Achtenberg, *Women as Healers* (Boston: Shambhala, 1991), 313.
6. Michael Castleman, *The Healing Herbs* (New York: Bantam, 1995), 18;

also Barbara Griggs, *Green Pharmacy* (Rochester, VT: Healing Arts Press, 1981), 144–46.

7. Lord Platt, "Medical Science: Master or Servant?" *British Medical Journal* 4, 439–44.
8. Castleman, *The Healing Herbs,* 11.

Chapter 4: HRT: The Road to the Present Dilemma

1. *Dorland's Medical Dictionary* (Philadelphia: W. B. Saunders, 1994), 776.
2. Sandra Coney, *The Menopause Industry* (Alameda, CA: Hunter House, 1994), 183–84.
3. Bernard Asbell, *The Pill* (New York: Random House, 1995), 86.
4. Barbara Griggs, *Green Pharmacy* (Rochester, VT: Healing Arts Press, 1981), 263.
5. Robert Wilson, *Feminine Forever* (New York: M. Evans and Company, 1966).
6. H. K. Ziel and W. D. Finkle, "Increased Risk of Endometrial Carcinoma among Users of Conjugated Estrogens," *The New England Journal of Medicine* 293, no. 23 (December 4, 1975): 1167–70.
7. John Lee, *What Your Doctor May* Not *Tell You About Menopause* (New York: Warner Books, 1996), 92. Dr. Lee establishes a Mayo Clinic conference in 1977 as the beginning point in the decision to add a progestin to conjugated estrogen, if a woman had a uterus, as protection against endometrial cancer.
8. U. Ottoson, et al., "Subfractions of high-density lipoprotein cholesterol during estrogen replacement therapy: A comparison between progestogens and natural progesterone," *Journal of Obstetrics and Gynecology* 151 (1985): 746–50.
9. Lee, *What Your Doctor May Not Tell You About Menopause,* 88.
10. Sandra Coney, *The Menopause Industry* (Alameda, CA: Hunter House, 1994), 202.
11. Information about horse farms provided by P.E.T.A.

Chapter 5: The Risk/Benefit Factor

1. Graham A. Colditz, Susan E. Hankinson, et al., "The use of estrogens and progestins and the risk of breast cancer in postmenopausal women," *The New England Journal of Medicine* 332, no. 24 (June 15, 1995): 1589–93.
2. Alan Gaby, "Research Review," *Nutrition & Healing,* March 1995, 7. Dr. Gaby was the questioner.
3. "Vital Signs," UCLA Medical Center newsletter, vol. 10 (August 1995): 4.
4. Ibid.; and Judith M. E. Walsh, "Cholesterol Screening in Young Adults," *Journal of the American Medical Association* 270, no. 13 (October 6, 1993): 1546(2).
5. Gaby, "Research Review," 7.
6. K. Randerson, "Cardiology Update, Garlic and the Healthy Heart," *Nursing Standard* 7, no. 30 (April 14–20, 1993): 51.
7. K. Dalery, et al., "Homocysteine and coronary artery disease in

French Canadian subjects; relation with vitamins B_{12}, B_6, pyridoxal phosphate, and folate," *American Journal of Cardiology* 75, no. 16 (June 1, 1995): 1107–11.

8. L. H. Kushi, et al., "Dietary antioxidant vitamins and death from coronary heart disease in postmenopausal women," *New England Journal of Medicine* 334, no. 18 (May 2, 1996): 1156–62.
9. Nancy E. Davidson, "Hormone Replacement Therapy—Breast versus Heart versus Bone," *New England Journal of Medicine* (June 15, 1995): 1638.
10. Ibid., 1638.
11. Lisa Seachrist, "What risk hormones?" *Science News* 148, no. 6 (August 5, 1995).
12. Aaron Folsom, et al., "Hormonal replacement therapy and morbidity and mortality in a prospective study of postmenopausal women," *American Journal of Public Health* 85, no. 8 (August 1995): 1128(5).
13. Quoted from a letter, circulated among colleagues but never printed, from Dr. Joel Hargrove and associates to *The New England Journal of Medicine.*

Chapter 6: More Than an Alternative

1. Bernard Asbell, *The Pill* (New York: Random House, 1995), 82–113.
2. Ibid., 82–113.
3. Ibid., 82–113.
4. Ibid., 82–113.
5. Ibid., 82–113.
6. Sandra Coney, *The Menopause Industry* (Alameda, CA: Hunter House, 1994), 185.
7. Information obtained from the International Academy of Compounding Pharmacists.
8. Per Bill Conway, product manager at the Berlichem division of Schering-Plough.
9. Barbara Griggs, *Green Pharmacy* (Rochester, VT: Healing Arts Press, 1981), 327–36.
10. Egon Diczfalusy, "The Early History of Estriol," *Journal of Steroid Biochemistry* 20, no. 48 (1984): 945–53.
11. AP Healthwire—January 24, 1996, Columbia Industries press release announcing release of Crinone.
12. Interviews with compounding pharmacists conducted from November 1995 through 1996.

Chapter 7: "The Naturals": What Are My Choices?

1. *Drug Facts and Comparisons,* 1996, p. 96.
2. 1996 *Physician's Desk Reference,* p. 2636. Indications and usage for Provera.
3. The Writing Group for the PEPI Trial, "Effects of Estrogen or Estrogen/Progestin on Heart Disease Risk Factors in Postmenopausal Women: The Postmenopausal Estrogen/Progestin Interventions

(PEPI) Trial," *Journal of the American Medical Association* 273, no. 3 (January 18, 1995): 199–208.
4. Ibid., 199–208.
5. Jerilynn C. Prior, et al., "Progesterone and the prevention of osteoporosis," *Canadian Journal of Obstetrics/Gynecology & Women's Health Care* 3 (1991): 178–84. Also, Jerilynn C. Prior, "Progesterone as a bone-trophic hormone," *Endocrine Reviews* 11 (May 1990): 386–98.
6. King-Jen Chang, et al., "Influences of percutaneous administration of estradiol and progesterone on human breast eipthelial cell cycle in vivo," *Fertility and Sterility* 63 (April 1995): 785–91.
7. J. F. DeBold and C. A. Frye, "Progesterone and the neural mechanisms of hamster sexual behavior," *Psychoneuroendocrinology* 19 (1994): 563–66.
8. Per Uzzi Reiss, M.D. These are Dr. Reiss's experiences with his patients.
9. Joel Hargrove, et al., "Menopausal hormone replacement therapy with continuous daily oral micronized estradiol and progesterone," *Obstetrics and Gynecology* 73, no. 4 (April 1989): 606–12. In addition, a follow-up study following women for five years is soon to be published and will confirm the results of this study.
10. Henry M. Lemon, et al., "Reduced estriol excretion in patients with breast cancer prior to endocrine therapy," *Journal of the American Medical Association* 196 (1996): 1128–34.
11. Alvin Follingstad, "Estriol, the forgotten estrogen," *Journal of the American Medical Association* 239, no. 1 (January 2, 1978): 29–30.
12. Walter E. Stamm and Raul Raz, "A controlled trial of intravaginal estriol in postmenopausal women with recurrent urinary tract infections," *New England Journal of Medicine* 329, no. 11 (September 9, 1993): 753–56.
13. Ibid.
14. Ibid.
15. Alvin Follingstad, "Estriol, the forgotten estrogen?" *Journal of the American Medical Association* 239, no. 1 (January 2, 1978): 29–30.

Chapter 8: Talking to Your Doctor About "The Naturals"

1. John Lee, M.D., *Natural Progesterone: The Multiple Roles of a Remarkable Hormone* (Sebastopol, CA: BLL Publishing, 1989), 89–90.
2. P. Hilts, "Dangers of some new drugs go undetected, study says," *The New York Times,* May 27, 1990.
3. "Drug R & D costs doubled in decade," *American Medical News* (May 18, 1990): 3, 53.
4. Geoffrey Redmond, *The Good News About Women's Hormones* (New York: Warner Books, 1995), 478–79.
5. Gail Sheehy, *New Passages* (New York: Random House, 1995), 219–20.
6. Carol Landau, Michele Cyr, and Anne Moulton, *The Complete Book of Menopause* (New York: Grosset/Putnam, 1994), 141.
7. Sheehy, *New Passages,* 201.

8. Chip Brown, "The Experiments of Dr. Oz," *The New York Times Magazine,* July 30, 1995, p. 2.

Chapter 9: Following the Natural Woman Plan

1. Sandra Coney, *The Menopause Industry* (Alameda, CA: Hunter House, 1994), 72.
2. Greer, *The Change,* 203.
3. Peter Ellison, et al., "The ecological content of human ovarian function," *Human Reproduction* 8, no. 12 (1993): 2248–58; also Ellison, "Measurements of salivary progesterone," *Annals of the New York Academy of Science* 694 (September 20, 1993): 161–76.
4. Jerilynn Prior, et al., "Reversible luteal phase changes and infertility associated with marathon training," *Lancet* 1 (1992): 269–70.
5. Lee, *What Your Doctor May* Not *Tell You About Menopause,* 110.
6. Winnifred B. Cutler, *Hysterectomy: Before and After* (New York: Harper & Row, 1988).
7. Elizabeth Vliet, "New Insights on Hormones and Mood," *Menopause Management,* Carrington Communications (June/July 1993): 140–46.

Chapter 10: How to Use "The Naturals"

1. Michael Murray, *The Healing Power of Herbs* (Rocklin, CA: Prima Publishing, 1995), 375.
2. Joel Hargrove, et al., "Menopausal hormone replacement therapy with continuous daily oral micronized estradiol and progesterone," *Journal of Obstetrics and Gynecology* 73 (October 1989): 606.
3. Katharina Dalton, *Once a Month* (Claremont, CA: Hunter House, 1990).
4. Lila Nachtigall, *Estrogen: The Facts Can Change Your Life* (Los Angeles: The Body Press, 1986), 51.
5. An interview conducted by C. Conrad with Dr. Jamie Grifo, 1995.

Chapter 11: Hormone Balancing Through Food

1. Nancy Beckham, "Phyto-oestrogens and compounds that affect oestrogen metabolism—Part I," *Australian Journal of Medical Herbalism* 7, no. 1 (1995): 10–16.
2. From an interview with Dr. John Potter in *Nutrition Action Health Letter,* April 1994, published by the Center for Science in the Public Interest.
3. Lee, *What Your Doctor May* Not *Tell You About Menopause,* 233.
4. "Soybeans show promise in cancer prevention," *Primary Care & Cancer* 15, no. 3 (March 1995): 11–12.
5. AP Newswire, April 16, 1996, on a study at the Department of Nutrition and Dietetics at King's College, London.
6. S. Barnes, et al., "Rationale for the use of genistein-containing soy matrices in chemoprevention trials for breast and prostate cancer," *Journal of Cellular Biochemistry* Supplement 22 (1995): 181–87.
7. Ibid., 181–87.
8. Herman Adlercreutz, et al., "Urinary excretion of lignans and

isoflavonoid phytoestrogen in Japanese men and women consuming a traditional Japanese diet," *American Journal of Clinical Nutrition* 54 (1991): 1093–1100.

Chapter 12: The Natural Woman Eating Plan

1. Marian Burros, "Developing a taste for organic milk," *The New York Times*, October 30, 1996, p. B4.
2. This information comes from reports prepared by the U.S. Department of Agriculture, and from articles by John Weihrauch and John Gardner, "Sterol content of foods of plant origin," *Journal of the American Dietetic Association* E73 (1979): 39–47; Nancy Beckham, "Phyto-oestrogens and compounds that affect oestrogen metabolism—Part I," *Australian Journal of Medical Herbalism* 7, no. 1 (1995): 10–16.
3. L. Kampf, "Treasures from the sea," *Delicious* (July 1996): 38–42.

Chapter 14: Taking Care of Your Bones

1. J. M. Riffee, *American Pharmacist* NS32, no. 8 (1992): 61–72.
2. *Stand up to Osteoporosis,* The National Osteoporosis Foundation, Washington, D.C., 1994.
3. Herman Aldercreutz, et al., "Urinary excretion of lignans and isoflavanoid phytoestrogen in Japanese men and women consuming a traditional Japanese diet," *American Journal of Clinical Nutrition* 54 (1991): 1093–1100.
4. C. Christiansen, et al., "Bone mass in postmenopausal women after the withdrawal of oestrogen/progestagen therapy," *Lancet* (February 29, 1981): 459–61; and D. T. Felson, et al., "The effect of postmenopausal estrogen therapy on bone density in elderly women," *The New England Journal of Medicine* 329 (1993): 1141–46.
5. John Lee, "Is natural progesterone the missing link in osteoporosis prevention and treatment?" *Medical Hypotheses* 35 (1991): 316–18; and "Osteoporosis reversal with transdermal progesterone," letter, *Lancet* 336 (1990): 1327.
6. Jerilynn Prior, "Progesterone as a bone-trophic hormone," *Endocrine Review* 11 (1990): 386–98.
7. William Regelson, *The Super-Hormone Promise* (New York: Simon & Schuster, 1996), 186.
8. J. S. Tenover, "Effects of testosterone supplementation in the aging male," *Journal of Clinical Endocrinological Metabolism* 75 (1990): 1092–95.
9. S. Rozenbergy, et al., "Age, steroids and bone mineral content," *Maturatis* 12 (1990): 137–143.
10. B. E. C. Nordin, et al., "The relation between calcium absorption, serum dehydroepiandrosterone, and vertebral mineral density in postmenopausal women," *Journal of Clinical Endocrinological Metabolism* 60 (1985): 651–57.
11. Ibid., 78.

12. H. Nawata, S. Tanaka, et al., "Aromastase in bone cell; association with osteoporosis in postmenopausal women," *Journal of Steroid Biochemistry Molecular Biology* 53, no. 1–6 (June 1995): 165–74.
13. Piet De Groen, et al., "Esophagitis associated with the use of aledronate," *New England Journal of Medicine* 335, no. 14 (October 3, 1996): 1016–21.
14. G. E. Abraham and H. Grewal, "A total dietary program emphasizing magnesium instead of calcium," *Journal of Reproductive Medicine* 35, no. 5 (1990): 503–7.
15. M. H. Knapen, K. Hamulyak, and C. Vermeer, "The effect of vitamin K supplementation on circulating osteocalcin (bone Gla protein) and urinary calcium excretion," *Annals of Internal Medicine* 111, no. 12 (1989): 100–5.

Chapter 15: An Ideal Way to Exercise

1. Leslie Bernstein, et al., "Physical excercise and reduced risk of breast cancer in young women," *Journal of the American Cancer Institute* 86, no. 18 (September 21, 1994): 1403–8.
2. Jane E. Brody, "Strength workouts, the training trend of the '90s, can help slow the ticking biological clock," *The New York Times,* August 10, 1994, pp. B6, C8.
3. Ibid., C8.
4. Ibid., C8.
5. Miriam Nelson, et al., "Effects of high density strength training on multiple risk factors for osteoporotic fractures: A randomized controlled trial." *Journal of the American Medical Association* 272, no. 24 (December 28, 1994): 1909–14.

Appendix D: Traditional Herbal Remedies

1. J. Chen, "Pharmacologic actions and therapeutic uses of ginseng and tang kwei," *International Journal of Chinese Medicine* 1, no. 3 (1984): 23–27.
2. W. Martin, "The miracle of evening primrose oil," *Townsend Letter for Doctors* (November 1992): 990–92.
3. M. Ishihara, "Effects of gamma-oryzanol on serum lipid peroxide levels and clinical symptoms of patients with climacteric disturbances," *Asia-Oceanic Journal of Obstetric Gynaecology* 10, no. 3 (1984): 317.
4. N. R. Kavinsky, "Vitamin E and the control of climacteric symptoms," *American Western Medicine and Surgery* 4, no. 1 (1950): 27–32.

INDEX